The Great Life Diet

A PRACTICAL GUIDE TO
Health, Happiness,
AND Personal Fulfillment

Denny Waxman

•

PREFACE BY MICHIO KUSHI

PEGASUS BOOKS
NEW YORK

THE GREAT LIFE DIET

Pegasus Books LLC
45 Wall Street, Suite 1021
New York, NY 10005

First Pegasus Books edition March 2007

Library of Congress Cataloging-in-Publication Data is available.

ISBN: 978-1-933648-26-2 36525771

10 9 8 7 8 6 5 4 3 2 1   "/67

Printed in the United States of America
Distributed by Consortium

PREFACE
BY MICHIO KUSHI

Humanity faces unparalleled opportunities and challenges as the new century unfolds. The world is unified more than ever through the Internet, cell phones, and other new technologies. At the same time, the threat of terrorism and nuclear blackmail, the outbreak of new viral diseases and epidemics, and the spread of cancer, heart disease, and other chronic ills are at an all-time high. Our children and grandchildren may inherit a globally warmed planet that is difficult to inhabit.

For the last half-century, macrobiotics has been in the forefront of the movement to promote personal and planetary health and peace. Derived from the traditional Greek words for "great life," macrobiotics encourages people to take responsibility for their own health and happiness by harmonizing with nature and the cosmos. The most effective way to do this is to eat a balanced natural foods diet, centered on whole grains, vegetables, beans, sea vegetables and fruits in harmony with the seasons, the climate, and other environmental factors.

The value of this approach is now almost universally accepted. In its food guidelines for the American people, the U.S. government officially promotes whole grains as the foundation of a healthy diet. The newest version of the Food Guide Pyramid, released in 2005, calls for brown rice, millet, whole wheat, and other grains to be the center of every meal.

The benefits of a macrobiotic diet are becoming increasingly recognized. At Harvard Medical School, cardiovascular researchers report that people eating a macrobiotic diet for an average of two years have virtually no risk of coronary heart disease, the major cause of death in modern society. Scientists at Tulane University in New Orleans, Louisiana, and the National Tumor Institute in Milan, Italy, report that a macrobiotic diet may help prevent or control cancer. Researchers at the New England Medical Center in Boston report that macrobiotic women process estrogen better than others and this may explain their low incidence of breast cancer. The National Cancer Institute wishes to start clinical trials on the macrobiotic approach to cancer after reviewing several of 76 medically-documented recoveries compiled by researchers for the National Institutes of Health.

Other medical studies have shown that a macrobiotic way of eating is beneficial for improving childhood nutrition, reducing violent and aggressive behavior among young juvenile offenders, controlling T-cells in young adults with AIDS, improving geriatric and psychiatric health, and reducing multiple chemical sensitivities.

According to environmentalists, a macrobiotic-oriented diet will benefit the earth as well as the people it sustains. Organically growing grains and vegetables as our staple crops instead of animal foods reduces our dependence on fossil fuels, chemicals, and other toxins, enriches the fertility of the soil, and results in cleaner air and water.

Over the years, Denny Waxman has been one of my closest students and associates and has served in the forefront of this health revolution. He founded Essene, the pioneer natural foods store in Philadelphia, in the late 1960s and organized seminars on diet and health in the 1970s. In the early 1980s, he helped Anthony J. Satillaro, M.D., the president of Methodist Hospital in Philadelphia, recover from terminal cancer. The story was featured in the *Saturday Evening Post*, *Life Magazine*, and later in a best selling book *Recalled by Life* and has helped to popularize macrobiotics around the world. At the Strengthening Health Institute that he founded in the 1990s, Denny has developed a simple, practical approach to macrobiotic education that focuses on seven steps to better health.

In *The Great Life Diet*, Denny distills the essence of macrobiotic principles and teachings. He presents his seven steps in a clear, concise way that can be readily understood and practiced. Seasoned with insights and humor from his personal experience, counseling practice, and global travels, the book offers a compass to maintaining health, happiness, and freedom. A wealth of practical information, including lists of recommended foods, basic recipes, and meal suggestions, helps the reader get started.

Thanks to Denny and a remarkable generation of macrobiotic teachers, counselors, and natural foods cooks, the seeds of a healthy, peaceful world community have been planted. *The Great Life Diet* is a passport to a healthier, more harmonious life.

MICHIO KUSHI
Brookline, Massachusetts

Michio Kushi is the leader of the international macrobiotic community. The Smithsonian Institution recognized his pioneering contribution to the modern organic, natural foods movement; complementary and alternative medicine; and peace education by establishing a permanent Kushi Family Collection on Macrobiotics at the National Museum of American History in Washington, D.C.

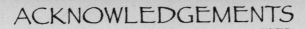

ACKNOWLEDGEMENTS

This book represents a major portion of my life. I would like to thank and acknowledge all the people who have helped me and are, therefore, a part of it.

Without my parents, Anna and Herman Waxman, I would not be able to offer this book. It is with the deepest respect and appreciation that I acknowledge them.

To Michio and Aveline Kushi, my spiritual parents, who have spent their lives teaching macrobiotics and spreading it throughout the world. They have given me endless inspiration, encouragement and personal guidance.

To my teachers, George and Lima Ohsawa, Herman and Cornelia Aihara, Shizuko Yamamoto, and William Dufty, who have dedicated their lives to macrobiotics and given us this powerful legacy.

To Takashi Yoshikawa, who has helped me so greatly to broaden and deepen my understanding of ki, which I have used to strengthen the health and lives of all those I have been privileged to help.

To my brother, Howard, who has shared the dream of macrobiotics and Essene with me.

To my children, Nathan, Joe, Naomi, Alisa, Madeline, Amy, Zoe, Andrew, Natasha, and Sam, who brighten my life.

To my friends and associates, Bill Tara, Murray Snyder, Bill Spear, Judith Flohr, Melanie Waxman, Michel Matsuda, Patrick Riley, Michel Abehsera, Michael Kessler, Gary Flaxenburg, and Gabor Szalontay, Rod and Peggy House, and Simon and Dragana Brown, with whom I have shared many macrobiotic adventures.

To my dear friends, Doug FitzSimons, Don and Mary Marti, Mona Schwartz and Helen Stevenson, who have played a very significant role in my life.

To Ruth Ann and Jeffrey Dubb, who opened their home to me and helped me on my return from Portugal.

To my dear friends and close associates at the SHI, Leslie Frodema, Warren Kramer, Michelle Nemer, Joe Waxman, Lear Blitzstein and Jeremy and Susan Higa, without whom my dream of building a school could not have been realized.

To Tara Gartner, for this beautifully designed book.

To Ellen Brodkey, my close and endearing friend, who has worked long and hard to make this book possible.

To my many other friends, too numerous to name, but you know who you are and I thank you.

And, finally, to my wife, Susan, who shares my life and my dreams.

TABLE OF CONTENTS

FOREWORD

*"Take care of your body with steadfast fidelity.
The soul must see things through these eyes alone,
and if they are dim, the whole world is clouded."*
—*Johann Wolfgang Von Goethe*

This book represents more than three decades of my life. Since I first tasted brown rice in 1967, I have been committed to understanding the principles of macrobiotics through study, practice, counseling and teaching. I have used the profound wisdom contained in these principles to transform my own life, to help raise healthy children, to guide thousands of clients back to health and to improve the health of countless others who have attended my seminars over the years. My goal has been, and continues to be, to find new ways to simplify and clarify these fundamental principles so they can be understood easily and practiced accurately by anyone interested in this way of life. Good health is our birthright and our heritage and ought to be available to everyone.

People want better health but they don't know how to achieve it. There is simply too much information available and it changes at too rapid a pace to be reliable. What's worse, this information, on which many people base their health practices, often turns out to be conflicting.

We can all make better choices every day, under any circumstances, if we understand what constitutes a good choice. The Strengthening Health Approach to Macrobiotics, which stresses an orderly approach to eating and living, is based on creating good eating habits, healthy food choices, and a way of life that nourishes the spirit. This book came into existence because of the frustration I felt at seeing people make often heroic efforts to improve their health yet not achieve the hoped for results. I have tested and observed the value of the Strengthening Health principles over many years and I am no longer amazed when I see a person change dramatically after just a month or two of following these principles. I hope you will make these principles a part of your life in the spirit of joy and adventure. Allow common sense to guide you. Observe the benefits that come from your practice. Should you find you are not getting the desired results, adjust what you are doing. Talk to those who have more experience and who can guide you. Try to proceed in the spirit of the early explorers who left the old ways behind in their search for greater freedom and richer lives. If you can do this, you will discover a quality of health that is life changing. Please use it well and share it with others.

INTRODUCTION

February 10, 1969 was the turning point of my life. It was the first day of my macrobiotic practice. A lot has happened since that day; a lot had happened before that day. I'd like to tell you about some of it.

I didn't embark on this way of life because of illness or because I saw it as a way of increasing my energy but because I was dissatisfied with my life. I had always had more than enough energy, perhaps too much, and my head was filled with ideas. My problem was figuring out what to do with all that vitality and all those ideas—in other words, what to do with my life.

I was graduated from high school in 1967, at the age of seventeen. Rather than work at a job I knew I wouldn't enjoy I decided to try college. Six months into the first semester I found my classes so boring and so meaningless that I dropped out to study on my own. That plan didn't work out either. The books I read depressed me even more. Many of them spoke of the glorious life and greatly enhanced abilities you could achieve through the development of your consciousness. Though their approaches differed, on one point the authors were all in agreement. In order to move in this direction, a teacher was required. But none of these books told me where to find one.

It was during this somewhat dark and restless period of my life that I first heard the word "macrobiotics." A friend's older brother used it in the process of describing a way of getting high by eating just brown rice. Of course, that is hardly what macrobiotics is all about but it caught my attention because of my own disastrous diet. I was a junk food addict. I ate meat only if it was between two slices of bread and I hated vegetables. I lived on sandwiches, pizza, cookies, candy, cake and soft drinks. Breakfast was my most substantial meal of the day and it consisted of a toasted bagel with butter and a coke. I will say, in my defense, that around this time I did notice that I was eating more and more junk food and feeling less and less satisfied—so the thought of eating brown rice and feeling better was quite appealing. Eager as I was to learn more about macrobiotics, no one I asked could tell me anything. My own stubbornness made me persist in the search and, eventually, a book appeared that would change my life.

The Unifying Principle

I came home one day to a house I shared with a group of friends in Philadelphia, to find a copy of "You Are All Sanpuku," by George Ohsawa, the 'father' of macrobiotics, on my bed. To this day, I have no idea how it got there. The book, which has an extensive introduction by William Dufty, one of Ohsawa's star students, transported me. It was the first book I'd ever read from beginning to end in one sitting and everything I had been searching for was in it. Ohsawa believed that we have the capacity to change our lives—that it is out of our daily diet and life style, things over which we have some measure of control, that we create our lives, for better or worse.

Ohsawa's book introduced me to the ancient eastern concept of Yin Yang, the principle of balance, harmony and change. He called it the "unique" or "unifying principle" because it explained both the unity and diversity of all things. In the eastern way of thinking, all of life has this dual nature.

I was more than ready to try something new. I went out the next day and bought brown rice, sea salt, mu tea (a kind of eastern herbal drink) and rushed home to cook my first meal. The taste was interesting—not good, not bad—but I felt wonderful and inspired. And so it was that I began my first 10-day rice fast as described by Ohsawa in his book. I didn't know it at the time but this was also the beginning of a new and wonderful life. Nor did I know I was having my first lesson in the unifying principle. And I most certainly didn't know that trouble was on the way.

The third day of my new regimen found me in the supermarket buying a half-gallon of ice cream, a box of graham crackers and a quart of orange juice. By the time I reached the checkout counter, I'd eaten most everything in the cart. To say that I was disappointed and confused is to understate the case. I knew in my heart that this philosophy and way of life were what I had been looking for—but, obviously, the diet was impossible. I had to find someone who knew more about macrobiotics.

As luck would have it, one day while I was having lunch in a health food store, a guy with a very intense look about him walked in. For some reason, I thought he might be macrobiotic and I was right. He told me he had come to Philadelphia to change the consciousness level of the city by opening a macrobiotic restaurant and that, yes, he was open to having a partner. A few days later, Stanley and I leased space in an underground mall called Sansom Village. That was on February 10, 1969.

Shortly afterwards, Stanley introduced me to Rod and Peggy House, two of Philadelphia's early macrobiotic friends, who gave me some invaluable dietary advice. The first thing they did was to suggest that I eat vegetables along with my brown rice, a change that made all the difference. That night, I ate my last steak sandwich and made my personal vow to practice the macrobiotic diet. With the help and guidance of Rod and Peggy, I found the diet easy to follow and the food delicious and satisfying. What I learned from my earlier, unsuccessful attempt to change my diet became the central point of what I would teach others—the importance of flexibility and common sense coupled with the understanding that change can happen gradually or it can happen in a flash.

A few days after we signed the lease, Stanley and I learned that the space wasn't zoned for a restaurant, which forced us to change our plans. We decided instead to open a food market with a lunch counter. We called it Essene Macrobiotic Supply. Shortly before the store opened, Michio Kushi, a world-renowned authority on macrobiotics and a former student of George Ohsawa's, came to Philadelphia to give a two-day seminar. I was one of the two hundred and seventy five people who had gathered to greet him and when I asked if he had any advice for our store he said, "Keep it clean. If it's not clean, it's not macrobiotic. I have seen many stores and restaurants that are not macrobiotic although they claim to be."

I couldn't believe that these were his words of wisdom. Keep it clean? Once again, I didn't understand the importance of what I was hearing. But I kept the store clean and over the years when people would comment on its cleanliness and tell me how wonderful it was to shop in such a place, I would thank them and think of Michio with gratitude.

We opened to the public on March 21, 1969 with six different products on the shelves, all of them in brown paper bags. People thought we were selling dog-food. We weren't disheartened. We continued to sell packaged grains from the shelves, adding some prepared food at the counter—cooked brown rice, miso soup, sauteed vegetables, raw salad, home-baked bread with apple or peanut butter, organic apple juice, fresh carrot juice and bancha tea.

Apparently, customers liked what we had to offer. They returned bringing friends. Business grew and we were able to fill the shelves with a variety of products. Our customers were curious. They wanted to know more about this mysterious food and the philosophy behind it. I told them about the wonders of eating grains and vegetables and about the harm that animal food, dairy, sugar and refined foods were inflicting on their bodies and minds. Some were interested; others were not and left. I decided to stop talking before we lost them all! Something good came out of this, however. I noticed that our regular customers began to change. They looked different—fresher, younger, more attractive. And these changes happened in a very short time.

Personal Changes and Studies

I was changing too. I had even more energy than before, even though my workday was very long and physically arduous. And I found I needed only five hours of sleep a night. I fell asleep quickly and awoke easily—just as George Ohsawa had said in his book. I was the cook and the baker. Every night at home, I prepared the sourdough bread and left it to rise in the heater. Every morning, at a little past five a.m., I baked the bread, prepared the day's food and transported it to the store. The food was kept warm in double boilers on electric hot plates.

Four changes convinced me of the personal benefits of my macrobiotic practice. First, I began to thoroughly enjoy grains and vegetables—and to feel satisfied by them. Remember that this discovery followed years of my refusing to eat vegetables or anything resembling "real food." My mother had had to strain the vegetables out of my soup before I would consider eating it! Once I began to appreciate vegetables, my incessant craving for junk food faded. The more macrobiotic food I ate, the more I enjoyed it. This was a revelation to someone with a history of always looking for his next snack.

Second, after several months of macrobiotic practice, I noticed that my libido and sexual vitality were increasing. I can't say I'd really noticed a decline, since it had occurred gradually over a period of a few years, but apparently my junk food diet and abusive life style had weakened me more than I'd realized.

The third change, though, was the most significant. Through macrobiotics, I discovered my direction in life. The future was filled with meaning. Each day was an adventure. I no longer counted the hours until I could go home as I'd done in every job I'd ever held until then.

And, fourth, I was able, finally, to see the value and power in my own life. When I was growing up, I was full of admiration for nearly everyone else. I believed everyone had better qualities or a better life than I. After practicing macrobiotics for a while, there came a day when I awoke thinking, "I'm glad I'm me." Somehow, I had gained confidence in myself and in my life. I felt refreshed and renewed. I could only attribute this profound change in outlook to my macrobiotic practice and study.

There were just two macrobiotic cookbooks at the time, Zen Cookery by George Ohsawa and Zen Macrobiotic Cooking by Michel Abehsera. I tried new recipes everyday. Cooking became an adventure. I was amazed and excited by how well the dishes turned out. Even non-macrobiotic friends liked them.

The store was my other big adventure. I looked forward to meeting the customers and seeing what they bought and what they ate. Talking with them and attempting to answer their questions, made me increasingly aware of my own lack of experience and understanding of macrobiotics. My dream was to study with Michio Kushi. Up to this point, my studies had been solely with Rod and Peggy House. Rod had given me my first shiatsu massage and had begun to teach me how to give shiatsu. (Shiatsu, a massage technique that uses finger pressure, has become widely accepted because of its effectiveness in dealing with a variety of common health problems.) Peggy had taught me to cook and both of them had encouraged me to stay in Philadelphia to develop Essene.

About a month after Essene opened, I visited one of Michio Kushi's study houses in Brookline, Massachusetts. Living in a study house seemed the best way to deepen my understanding of macrobiotics. It would also give me a chance to hear Michio speak. He lectured a few evenings a week and each lecture was a revelation. To witness his capacity for life, to receive the gift of his understanding of nature, the universe, health, science and history was mind altering. I couldn't get enough.

I decided to see Michio for a consultation. He invited me over at lunchtime and didn't stop eating while we talked. After some brief casual conversation, he looked at my palm and told me I was a hard worker. Then he drew the standard macrobiotic diet on a small piece of paper. I asked if I should eat fish. He said, "not much." I asked if there was anything else he had to tell me. He told me to eat miso soup every day. I prodded him some more. He told me about the special leadership seminar he was giving over the summer. I decided then and there to go even though Essene needed my attention.

"I have never let schooling interfere with my education."

—*Mark Twain*

Michio lectured nearly every day for three months during that summer. The topics included macrobiotic philosophy and cooking, shiatsu massage, Oriental diagnosis and medicine, meditation and other spiritual practices. I felt as if I had finally begun to practice macrobiotics. I had learned so much that was new and inspiring from Michio's lectures and from my stay in the study house. I returned to Philadelphia filled with the spirit of macrobiotics and eager to make Michio's teachings a part of my own life and to share them with others.

About six months after we opened Essene, Stanley disappeared and was never heard from again. So it was that when Rod and Peggy House left for Brookline, I became, by default, Philadelphia's macrobiotic leader. Although I was only twenty-one at that time, I was the person with the most experience in macrobiotic studies and practice. I began teaching immediately and within the year I was able to offer private counseling to clients.

Thirty-some years have passed since then and in all that time I have never stopped studying. The focus of my thinking has been and continues to be how best to apply the principles of macrobiotics to the daily strengthening of individual health.

How I discovered the Strengthening Health Approach

Over the years I've observed thousands of people practice macrobiotics—some with great success and some with none at all. I've spent a great deal of time trying to pinpoint the difference between a successful practice and a failed one.

Generally speaking, people who undertake the practice of macrobiotics fall into one of two groups: those interested in macrobiotics as a way of life and those interested in the diet. By and large, those drawn to the macrobiotic philosophy tend to approach macrobiotics with an open mind and a sense of excitement. They don't feel limited or restricted by the practice. On the contrary, they feel they have received the gift of freedom.

Those who come because of the diet, having heard that the diet is strict, limited and arduous tend, unfortunately, to model their practice along those lines. Unless the individuals in this group can learn to appreciate macrobiotics as a flexible, harmonious and satisfying way of life, they often have difficulty adapting to and staying with the practice.

After many years of counseling, I decided it was time to look at how macrobiotics was being presented to the world. My goal was to find a way to make macrobiotics more open and accessible to the general public. In 1992, in search of insight, my family and I moved to Portugal. We stayed three years. One beautiful day, while sitting on the beach gazing at the water and enjoying the sunshine, an idea came to me. Why not teach people how and what to add to their lives rather than focus on how and what to give up?

What is a macrobiotic diet anyway?

George Ohsawa introduced macrobiotics to the United States in 1950. He created 10 diets that you will find summarized in the following chart. His 10 diets ranged from No. 7, a diet consisting only of grains, down to No. −3, a diet consisting of 10% grains and 90% other foods. The numbering is purposeful and the number seven is especially significant. God created the earth in seven days; there are seven days in a week; seven is the number of orbits in a complete spiral.

Diet #	Grains	Vegetables	Soup	Animal	Salad/Fruit	Dessert
7	100%					
6	90%	10%				
5	80%	20%	10%			
4	70%	30%	10%			
3	60%	30%	10%			
2	50%	30%	10%	10%		
1	40%	30%	10%	20%		
-1	30%	30%	10%	20%	10%	
-2	20%	30%	10%	25%	10%	5%
-3	10%	30%	10%	30%	15%	5%

Doesn't the chart seem to imply that Diet No. 7 is the best one? That Diet No. 6 is not quite as good but still worthy? After all, we marvel at the beauty of six-sided figures like snowflakes or honeycombs. That Diet No. 5 is also appealing, a strong number calling to mind a pentagon? Don't the negative or minus numbers make us feel as if we are being penalized? If this is your thinking, you are not alone. Many people at one time or another have believed that Diet No.7, in its total devotion to grain, is the ideal.

Although I never met George Ohsawa, Michio and Aveline Kushi believe that his true intention was to show the variety possible in macrobiotic practice and not to rank the diets. Even though Ohsawa was incredibly diverse in his practice and lifestyle, many of those who followed his teachings were not. And, many of those who knew Ohsawa personally insist that his teachings alone are valid. He had a kind of power about him that captivated people.

The Kushi Standard Macrobiotic Diet

To dispel the notion that a macrobiotic diet demands adherence to a single plan, the Kushi's used another approach. They averaged Ohsawa's 10 diets to show the variety and flexibility available in macrobiotic practice. They created the Standard Macrobiotic Diet and made it easily accessible by presenting it as a pie divided into various sized slices.

- 40% to 60% cereal grains
- 1 to 2 bowls of soup
- 20% to 30% vegetables
- 5% to 10% beans and sea vegetables
- Other foods revolving around the main ones, including condiments, seasonings, nuts, seeds, fruits, sweets, desserts, white-meat fish and beverages

1-2 BOWLS OF VEGETABLE SOUP DAILY

with miso, shoyu or sea salt

40-60% WHOLE CEREAL GRAINS DAILY

Grains may be whole or cracked and in simple combinations, unyeasted sourdough breads, whole grain pastas, noodles or dumplings.

Eat cereal grains & grain products with every meal—breakfast, lunch & dinner

20-30% VEGETABLES DAILY

Vegetables may be boiled, steamed, sauteed, pressed, pickled, raw, etc.

Eat at least one vegetable dish with every meal.

5-10% BEANS, BEAN PRODUCTS & SEA VEGETABLES

Most people who encounter Ohsawa's standard diet in table form perceive it as rigid, limited and forbidding. When they see the Kushi's formulation—the pie shape—they envision a plate divided into portions—a visual representation of how a meal should look: here is the portion of grain, of soup, etc.

Without meaning to, both these approaches somehow give the impression that the goal is a perfect practice. They create the image that macrobiotics is about perfection. But it's always been my belief that the point of macrobiotics is to recreate ourselves each day as who we really want to be. To accomplish this, we must create an orderly life by learning how to make interesting, healthful choices. Perfection, even if there were such a thing, is irrelevant. What we are looking for is an orderly and balanced way of eating. Why? Because it is in the nature of things that balance craves more balance.

Food is our strongest desire. In a contest between a craving and an individual's willpower, the craving always wins. For example, if you consume enough salt you will feel thirsty and have to drink. If you eat dry toast regularly, sooner or later you will begin to crave something sweet or rich like butter or jam to put on it. If you resist the temptation, you will crave something even sweeter and richer later on. There is no exception. In the end, food always wins. Better to discard the notion that the macrobiotic diet demands perfect obedience. If you don't, trouble will follow.

Our second strongest desire is for sex. Few people can conquer the desire for sex. A strong desire can be suppressed, diminished or even lost because of declining health but the loss of desire usually has a harmful effect on the other parts of our lives.

It's easy to extend the idea that if perfection is possible in the areas of diet and sexual activity, it is also possible in other areas of life, in work, for instance, or in relationships. But this is a completely unrealistic concept and to guide our lives according to it would be supremely foolish and lead only to despair.

According to this kind of wrong-headed thinking, if we should eat something that doesn't fit with our notion of the perfect diet then we're no longer macrobiotic—the experiment is over. Now let's try a different way of looking at the subject: instead of worrying about giving up certain foods, instead of thinking, "no meat, no chicken, no eggs, no this, no that," why not consider adding foods. Ask yourself "what would be good for me to eat, what would I really like to eat, what will further my life?"

Don't take away anything. Start by adding grains to your present diet. To complement the grains, add vegetables. Follow that by adding soup. Finally, add other foods: beans, sea vegetables, white-meat fish, fruits, desserts and beverages. Where you stop adding is up to you. Do you want to stop with a completely vegetarian menu or do you want to include fish? The choice is yours. When you approach the subject this way, the likelihood of your wanting other animal food is remote. In my experience, most people lose their taste for animal and dairy food after they begin eating grains and vegetables. The rewards to mind and body are so enormous that we begin to crave the foods that provide the most benefit and the greatest sense of health and well being.

As soon as we are told not to have something, it seems we want it all the more. Prohibition increases desire. Whether we really desire it or not is hardly the point. Let me give you an example from my own life. I was never much of a fruit eater but on one particular day in Boston I ate a lot of it. That night, after Michio's lecture, when I went up to ask him a question, he replied only, "Too much fruit." However, in spite of his remark, for the next few weeks I ate more and more fruit. I couldn't stop. It was as if a dam had burst. I don't like fruit all that much and here I was going crazy over it.

Most people find it extremely difficult to give up their favorite foods. We spend our entire lives eating a particular way and even though we may know that the foods we love are making us sick, we cannot give them up without a struggle. Younger people often have a harder time than older ones, perhaps because many older people remember a more natural, orderly way of eating from their own childhood. Our memory for food is very strong and, as we age, our tastes are more likely to revert to the tastes we developed while we were growing up.

The insight I was looking for, the one that came to me that day on the beach in Portugal was this: Why not begin the practice of macrobiotics by adding healthy foods to the individual's current diet? Why take anything away? Wouldn't this approach help people switch to the macrobiotic diet at their own pace and with less difficulty? My observation since then has been that this approach works pretty well. From that day to this, my dream has been to continue finding new ways to make the practice and value of macrobiotics more open and accessible.

In the mid eighties, I had developed a program called Discovery that was designed to teach people everything they needed to know about macrobiotics in one day. I also incorporated a very abbreviated version of Discovery into my one hour counseling sessions. At the time, it was the only way I could think of to help my clients implement the major life-style changes I was recommending to them.

I devoted a five-minute portion of the Discovery program to making the transition to a healthier diet and life-style. I advised people on how to encourage family and friends to change their ways of eating. As a first step, I introduced them to healthier foods and life-style practices. At the same time, I urged them not to worry about giving up any of the foods they were attached to. But it was not until that day at the beach that I realized just how widely applicable the principle behind Discovery was. In fact, the Discovery Program proved to be the seed for this book.

On my regular trips back to the United States during the years I lived in Portugal, I lectured often on the Strengthening Health approach. I offered public seminars and a two-weekend-long course to train people in this approach. When I moved back to the States in 1995, I made a concentrated effort to introduce this approach to as many people as possible, an effort that continues to this day at The Strengthening Health Institute which was founded in 1997. The School of Strengthening Health and Macrobiotic Counseling is its educational arm and offers a number of different programs.

Many of the clients who seek my help come to me with serious illnesses, such as cancer and diabetes. Even so, I will sometimes recommend that they add healthier food to their diets before encouraging them to give up the foods they usually eat. With very few exceptions, they gravitate naturally toward the healthier food.

If we change our diet, even in a limited way, our food cravings change too. Many of us feel guilty or weak-willed if we can't stick to a specific diet. It's important to understand that by eating certain foods we set ourselves up for failure. Cravings are not a matter of mind control, discipline, or will power but are the expression of a mechanical process. Cravings are a manifestation of the body's desire for balance.

My point is this: if you approach the subject of eating healthfully in a positive manner by thinking of expanding your food choices rather than denying yourself the foods you crave, you are more likely to be successful. Start by selecting grains that satisfy and nourish you. Then choose vegetable dishes and other foods. Make these choices part of your daily meals and, at the same time, make daily exercise a habit. Finally, take a look at the other areas of your life and start to include things that can bring you to balance. After a short while you will begin to experience a kind of natural satisfaction. Then you can decide how much you want to do on a regular basis in the areas of diet and eating habits, exercise and life style. The choice is solely yours. Strengthening your health is an ongoing process.

This positive approach is the basic concept underlying The Great Life Handbook and it is a concept that is infinitely adaptable. For instance, you may choose to eat the best organically grown grains and grain products, or you may choose commercial whole wheat or rye bread or pasta as your grain product. This flexibility means that you may practice these principles in a diner, a deli, a fine restaurant, or at home.

The vegetables you select can be of the highest quality, organically grown from your own garden, freshly picked and prepared; or you can order conventionally grown steamed broccoli at an Italian restaurant or at a diner. The same principle applies to soup. The choice runs the gamut from the best homemade organic vegetable soup to jazzed-up canned soup. You may apply these principles across the board—wherever you find yourself. You can adjust food quality up or down as long as you keep to the format. You may use instant foods, microwave foods, restaurant and take out foods or you may choose to prepare the best home cooked food everyday. There are many options and many ways to apply the Strengthening Health principles to your own life. As you can see, what I'm really talking about here is a way of life, an approach to life. What The Great Life Handbook offers is an orderly approach to diet and lifestyle.

As with most things in life, perception often determines outcome. If you perceive macrobiotics as a closing spiral, one that narrows and limits you, you will most probably abandon it because you will find the practice too difficult and too rigid. If, on the other hand, you conceive of it as an opening spiral, one that expands your freedom and widens your thinking, you will be off on a fabulous lifelong adventure. Your vision and your approach are the catalysts to strengthening your health.

In formulating these ideas, I made a couple of conscious decisions. First, everything I had to say here would derive from collective human experience and wisdom. Second, everything would have a basis in common sense, one of the few qualities of mind I believe in strongly. Scientific theories come and go. Common sense, grounded in human experience, prevails over time. I think it's hard to fault the following seven step program. Try it out for a month or so and see for yourself.

THE SEVEN STEPS

> "Health is a state of complete physical, mental and social well-being, and not merely the absence of disease or infirmity."   —Heave

The Strengthening Health Method proposes an orderly approach to eating and living. It is based on creating healthy eating habits, a balanced diet, and beneficial lifestyle practices. With this in mind, let's get started on the 7 Steps.

> "Health, without which there is no happiness."
> —Thomas Jefferson

EATING HABITS: FORMAT OF MEALS

1. Take time for your meals everyday.

Sit down to eat your meals or snacks without doing other things.

Allow adequate time for your meals.

Eat slowly and chew well.

Stop eating three hours before bedtime.

Eat in an orderly manner.

Avoid mixing foods in the same mouthful.

2. Set your daily schedule.

Rise early and go to sleep before midnight.

Keep your mealtimes regular.

DIET: CONTENT AND QUALITY OF MEALS

3. Eat two or three complete and nutritionally balanced meals every day.

Plan every meal around cooked grains and grain products.

Complete and balance every meal with one to two vegetable dishes.

LIFESTYLE: APPROACH TO HEALTH

4. Make your daily life active.

Walk for thirty minutes every day.

Give yourself a daily body rub.

Life related exercise provides the most benefit for lasting health.

Cultivate and take time for hobbies.

5. Create a more natural environment.

Surround yourself with green plants especially in the bed room, the kitchen, the bathrooms and office or workspace.

Wear pure cotton clothing next to your skin.

Use natural materials such as wood, cotton, silk and wool in your home.

6. Make your macrobiotic practice work.

Keeping to the format of meals improves your ability to make healthier food choices.

Keep a daily record of your meals to help you become more objective about your practice.

7. Cultivate the spirit of health.

Be open, curious and endlessly appreciative of all of life.

Be flexible and adaptable in your practice.

Develop a strong will and the determination to create your own health.

Be accurate in your practice.

Create a good support network.

Learn to cook well.

> "Ill-health, of body or of mind, is defeat. Health alone is victory. Let all men, if they can manage it, contrive to be healthy."
>
> —*Thomas Carlyle*

The Origin of the Seven Steps

Where do the Seven Steps come from? In other words, what is the model on which they are based? The answer is simple. They are based on my observation of nature. If we observe nature closely over time, two clear patterns emerge. The first is that nature is orderly and consistent. As a result, its cycles are 100% predictable. For example, we know that the sun will rise and set everyday. We know the exact time at which this will happen. We know the exact position the sun will occupy in the sky at any given moment. We can predict where it will be at any time in the future. We can project backwards with the same certainty. The sun never takes a break, never takes a day off. If the sun fails to rise, either there is no more sun or our planet is out of orbit. Either way our worries will be over! We also know that every month, without exception, the moon will move from new to full and back again, as surely as we know that every year spring will follow winter and summer will follow spring. However, we can never be certain what any individual season, month, week, day or hour will be like. Sometimes May is atypically rainy and cold while June can be as hot as August. From this observation, we can conclude that nature is orderly and consistent while at the same time it is endlessly variable and inconsistent. These are nature's two patterns. Simple, yet it seems that in the practice of macrobiotics the two most difficult concepts to understand are those of balance and variety.

> "Common sense and nature will do a lot to make the pilgrimage of life not too difficult."
>
> —*W. Somerset Maugham*

Balance

If, as I am proposing, our sense of balance comes directly from nature then the easiest way to achieve balance is to align with nature's orderly cycles. To choose to align with endless variety, inconsistency and change is obviously to choose failure. But we can easily align with the very orderly aspects of nature—its cycles of sunrise, sunset, and seasons.

Variety

Let's take a look at the principle of variety as it applies to macrobiotics. In macrobiotics, we believe that everything has its complimentary opposite, some other aspect that completes it or brings it to wholeness or to oneness: day—night, man—woman, heat—cold, happiness—sadness, health—sickness, etc. This is true for nature as well. Its orderly cycles are complemented and completed by its cycles of endless variety, change and inconsistency. These are nature's two aspects or you might say nature's front and back. The point is that the way we can best align with nature's variety is through nature's orderly cycles. This is key to our understanding.

Appetite

With this in mind, I'd like to pose another basic question. Where does our appetite come from? What determines what our appetite is on any given day, month or year? Many years ago, when there were a number of macrobiotic study houses in Philadelphia and the community was very closely knit, on any given day you could be sure that almost exactly the same meal was being served in all the different locations—dish for dish, sometimes ingredient for ingredient. Why? We could, I suppose, blame it on gossip. The macrobiotic grapevine is amazingly efficient! However, these different study houses were not sharing menu plans. There is a principle at work behind the similarity and it is that the nature of each day calls for certain types of food, certain dishes. And so the people who were more aligned with nature were all drawn to the same foods. In other words, their appetites were aligned with nature and therefore with each other so that when they planned their meals they chose nearly identical foods and cooking styles.

Our appetite, our taste and sense of variety all come from nature. Now let me take this a step further. Some people argue that having a set schedule is too rigid a way to live. But if we look at nature it's hard to say that nature is rigid. Nature is full of change and inconsistency. Nature is asymmetrical and nature has no lack of vitality. If you cut things down, they will grow again.

Whatever we do to the earth, the earth has the ability to adjust, adapt, repair and maintain itself. Based on this observation, we can say that nature has great vitality.

"After you have exhausted what there is in business, politics, conviviality, and so on have found that none of these finally satisfy, or permanently wear what remains? Nature remains."

—*Walt Whitman*

Vitality

Where does this vitality come from? I have an answer that satisfies me. You might agree with it, you might not. I believe nature's vitality is the result of its orderliness. For example, if you grow up in an orderly family, one that has structure, routines and traditions, one that values consistency so that you know what to expect, then automatically you have a kind of confidence and a vitality for life. Whereas, if you grow up in a family where nothing is consistent and life is disorderly, you don't have that positive kind of vitality. Let's suppose, for the purpose of argument, that you have job security and that you know what's expected of you. In such a situation, you can work hard and efficiently without becoming exhausted. But if your job is in jeopardy from day to day and you're not sure what is expected of you exhaustion sets in almost automatically. Am I right? You lose your energy. You lose your vitality. You lose your creativity. Can you see the influence order and structure exert over our lives and health? Order and structure are what give us vitality, adaptability and creativity, confidence and a zest for life.

If you talk with very old people about their lives, you will discover that what most of them have in common is an orderly life. Set times for sleeping, waking and meals, times that don't vary. These people are self-sufficient. They rarely, if ever, see doctors. They prefer to guide their own lives and to take care of all their needs themselves. Generally, they live simply. And, because over the years they have maintained this orderliness, they have been rewarded with good health, strong vitality and long life.

Structure and creativity

I read about an experiment that was done some time ago that is pertinent to what we're talking about. The researchers asked a certain number of people who had had no previous experience in the field of advertising to come up with slogans for various products. The subjects were offered no guidelines whatsoever. The same thing was asked of computers but since computers can't function without being programmed the computers were given very clear guidelines. The results didn't surprise me although they may have surprised the researchers. The slogans the human subjects came up with were too boring and childish to attract any attention. The computers, on the other hand, produced highly creative material that was as good as any dreamt up by the world's most successful advertising agencies. The difference from the macrobiotic point of view was that the human subjects were given no guidelines, no structure, while the computers were given explicit instructions—this is what we want, this is what you may do, this is what you may not do. The point is that alignment with nature's orderly cycles is the key to understanding variety. It is the key that unlocks freshness and creativity.

Seven steps

Some of you may have seen the 7 Steps bookmark, all seven steps printed on a slender bookmark. When I lecture, I often say to people that now they know everything I know. People think I'm joking. I'm not. I'm very serious. If you do these things and bring yourself into alignment with nature, then you and I will be receiving life from the same source—including our appetite, food choices, ideas and understanding. We all have the ability to align with nature and its orderly cycles. All we need is the will and to be shown the way.

I hope that now you can appreciate why an explanation of Eating Habits: Format of Meals had to precede an exploration of the actual Diet: Content of Meals. Eating Habits are the controlling factor. The bottom line is that good eating habits create the ability to make healthy choices. Let's say I fill a table with the best quality and most delicious macrobiotic food and you eat nothing but food from that table. Will that be a guarantee of good health? I don't think so. You won't achieve good health until you learn how to choose the foods you need. We build our health one day at a time, one meal at a time. You must learn to choose appropriately.

The question is, of course, how do we do this? Again, the answer is by adhering to a structure, by incorporating the structure of the Seven Steps into our daily lives.

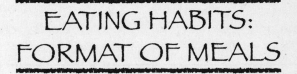

EATING HABITS:
FORMAT OF MEALS

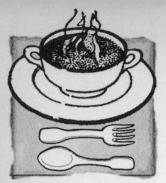

STEP 1

TAKE TIME FOR YOUR MEALS EVERYDAY

SIT DOWN TO EAT YOUR MEALS OR SNACKS WITHOUT DOING OTHER THINGS.

This is the first step towards good health and will help you feel more satisfied. Sitting down to eat is an expression of our appreciation and respect for our food. Sitting down enables us to create order in our daily eating habits and it makes us more conscious of what we eat. The tendency is not to count the food we eat while standing. It just doesn't enter our consciousness. In fact, we usually stand when eating the foods we really don't want to eat or shouldn't be eating. If you tend to snack through-out the day, you will have trouble regulating your meals and per-haps have some difficulty with weight control. Generally, we don't realize how much food we ingest when we are eating con-stantly. Remember that many people eat not because they are hungry but out of a desire to soothe their nerves or lessen their frustration. For them, food acts as a tranquilizer. If this is true in your case, you will become more aware of it if you sit down whenever you snack. You may even decide you don't really want to eat at that time.

Chinese medicine says that food has both physical aspects and chi (or energetic) aspects. If you want to absorb the ener-getic aspects of your food, your stomach must be in the bent position it takes when you are seated, not in the elongated posi-tion it assumes when you stand. As I see it, different positions are for different activities. Standing is for being active and productive; reclining, which is a receptive position, is for sleep, sex and rest; and sitting is a transitional position between the two postures. We eat during the day so that we have the energy to be active. We sleep at night so that the body, using the food consumed during the day, can repair and maintain itself.

> "If the soul is a kind of stomach, what is spiritual communion but an eating together?"
>
> —*Thomas Carlyle*

Sitting, standing and lying down

Sitting is the link between standing and lying down. Think about how the seated position aligns with eating. The seated position is the one in which the change between the external and internal environments, between giving out and taking in, occurs. Sitting is the position for receiving nourishment, for strengthening the ability to absorb, digest and assimilate food. It is also the position most congenial to the process of thinking. Try reading while standing up or lying down. Ideas are not as easily understood in these positions. Whether we are talking about absorbing, digesting and assimilating food or ideas, sitting is unique.

If you eat while standing up, your stomach cannot accept the food properly. Standing interferes with the digestive process. When you sit down to eat, you will be more conscious of what you are eating and also how much you are eating. Since sitting is a more relaxed position than standing, you will probably eat less food because you will be digesting what you have eaten more thoroughly and will be satisfied with smaller amounts. When you are seated and you overeat, often you don't know it until you get up from the table. Then you think—oh-oh, I ate too much. In other words, what you are experiencing at that moment of awareness is a natural sensation of fullness. This gives you a gauge by which to measure how much is too much. On the other hand, if you eat standing up you never know when you've had enough. You lose your natural sense of how much food it takes to satisfy you.

Eastern and western medicine

In the early stages of medicine, during the era of Hippocrates, eastern and western medicine were very similar. Both were grounded in practical knowledge and common sense. Both taught the importance of diet and life style in creating good health. In those days, health advice included instructions for properly handling all aspects of life. People were taught to sit up straight when eating and to chew their food thoroughly. These guidelines were considered rudimentary. Then as the East moved toward a more spiritual way of life and the West gravitated toward science and analysis, their commonly held ideas became increasingly divergent. However, certain of these ideas—like sitting down to eat and chewing properly—were passed on from one generation to the next in both the East and the West.

> "Tradition is a guide and not a jailer."
>
> —W. Somerset Maugham

Nourishment and balance

Ideally, a meal is a time for nourishing and balancing oneself. A meal is a time to be relaxed, open and receptive to nourishment and these attributes don't mix well with activity. Eating while doing other things such as reading, working, watching TV, talking on the phone, or driving interferes with your ability to receive nourishment. Light, quiet conversation is fine because it makes you more open and receptive. (Heavy, loud conversation tightens you up and closes you down.) My analogy is this: If we're talking and in the middle of our conversation I pick up a book, I close off to you. If you're eating, trying to receive nourishment from your food, and you do something else at the same time you close off to your food. It's that simple. You aren't being fully nourished. Each of us takes different nourishment from the same food. Our ability to receive nourishment depends on how we eat and on our approach to eating.

Many of us don't like to sit down and eat without doing other things, especially when we are alone. When we eat alone, what happens? Thoughts and feelings come up, memories come up.

Often we don't like what comes up but if we learn to think of this as part of a cleansing process, of getting things out that don't belong inside us, it should be easier to eat without distractions. And, if we can be patient and allow the unhappy thoughts and feelings to come up, they will be followed by happier ones. In the beginning, just try to let go of your thoughts as you would in meditation. Acknowledge each thought as it comes and then let it pass away.

Food is our strongest desire in life. Food also has the capacity to give us an incredibly deep sense of satisfaction. If we eat quietly and without distraction, we will feel deeply satisfied and fulfilled. However, many people don't allow this to happen. As soon as unhappy feelings come up, they automatically feel the need to do something, to jump up, to read something, to turn on the TV. It's very important to get past this. Let's say that when you begin to practice macrobiotics you abruptly stop drinking coffee. A headache follows. You can either allow the headache to pass (and the pain might be very intense for a few days) or you can drink a cup of coffee and end it. You might not think so but this situation is analogous to eating without doing other things. Eating while you distract yourself with something else is the same as taking the very thing (coffee) that was the cause of your problem (headache) in the first place. The cause is also the cure—albeit a very temporary one.

Of all my recommendations, I think sitting down to eat without doing other things is the most difficult one for my clients to practice. At the same time, it's the most important of all the steps. It's the one that sets our direction towards health or towards sickness.

Highlights:

- Sitting down to eat your meals and snacks without doing other things is the first step towards good health.

- When you eat without distraction, you absorb the most nutrition.

- You need to concentrate when you read a book or see a movie to get the most out of the experience. You need to participate fully in a conversation to be completely satisfied. This principle applies to your meals as well.

- Sitting down to eat without doing other things allows you to be more aware of what you are eating and to stop when you have had enough.

- You eat less and feel more satisfied.

- This is one of the most difficult steps. Try always to be conscious of it.

ALLOW ADEQUATE TIME FOR YOUR MEALS.

The minimum time required to consume a meal is twenty minutes. Now you might think that that's an arbitrary number, but it isn't. Let me explain. According to Eastern thinking, everything in the universe is energy, some of it materialized energy (us, for example) and some not (wind, for example). Energy is manifested in vibrations. And we know that vibrations have a natural tendency to align with each other—that's physics. I first realized this when I was in Switzerland, in a shop that sold cuckoo clocks. All the pendulums were exactly aligned. (I was so pleased with my discovery that I made the mistake of buying one of these clocks. It drove me crazy once I was home.) Or, take the example of women's menstruation. It's well known that after a short while women who share living quarters begin to menstruate at the same time. Therefore, it should not surprise you to learn that after twenty minutes in the same room the rate of heartbeat, blood pressure and breathing of those present tends to align. By the same token, if someone should enter the room whose rate of heartbeat, blood pressure or breathing is very different from that of the group's—too different for alignment to occur—everyone will feel some discomfort, no one will be able to relax completely. Understandably, the person who entered the room will feel too uncomfortable to stay very long.

Fifty cycles of energy every day

Why does the process of alignment take roughly twenty minutes? Here is the reasoning: fifty cycles of energy (ki, the Japanese word for energy) flow through the body each day. This means that ki circulates through the entire body fifty times a day. One cycle takes just under thirty minutes. It takes seventy percent of the thirty-minute cycle, or about twenty minutes, for alignment to become significant. You can check on this yourself. When you go somewhere new, how long does it take until you really feel comfortable? How long does it take to settle into a serious conversation? It takes about twenty minutes. Still, many people sit down to eat a meal assuming that five to ten minutes is an adequate amount of time. It certainly isn't. If a friend says he has something really important to talk over with you and you say—great, I can give you five minutes—it's likely he or she will feel insulted. You can't have a serious conversation in five minutes. You can introduce the subject but you can't delve into it. In the same way, you can have an appetizer or a snack in five minutes but not an entire meal.

Breakfast is the most forgiving meal because we're active for a full day afterwards. Dinner is the least forgiving. In other words, if you have a fifteen-minute breakfast, it's not the end of the world. But in a manner of speaking, a fifteen-minute dinner is. It doesn't count as a meal. I'm not talking about solid eating time. I'm talking about the time it takes to complete your meal—from the moment you sit down until the moment you get up from the table.

Let's say you're standing next to someone at a bar. Even if you don't say a word to that person, after twenty minutes your energy will be aligned. If you smile at that person, the alignment happens more quickly. If you talk together, it happens more quickly still and the alignment becomes stronger. I hope you can see now that quiet conversation during mealtimes, talking and eating together, fosters a strong and deep alignment. If you eat quietly without talking, you become more independent, but not as strongly connected to one another. Whether you eat alone or with others, the minimum time for a meal is twenty minutes.

Highlights:

- The minimum time for a meal is twenty minutes.

- Time yourself from the beginning to the end of the meal, not just while you are eating.

- Breakfast is the most forgiving meal in terms of time.

- It takes time for your body to adjust from being active to receiving nourishment just as it takes time to settle into a good conversation.

EAT SLOWLY AND CHEW WELL.

It's only common sense that in order to eat slowly you must be seated. You must also allow time in your mind for the meal. If you don't do this you won't be able to slow down. If, when you sit down, you are thinking that you're running late, that you don't have time for this meal, you won't be able to eat slowly. Once you pick up your fork, the pace is set and it's very hard to change it. In other words, eating slowly and chewing well require some preparation.

> "Chew your drink, and drink your food."
>
> —Mahatma Ghandi

Chewing and posture

In order to chew well, we have to assume the correct posture. The posture for chewing and the posture for reading are exactly the same. If you have something to read that is important to you and requires deep understanding, then you had better sit up straight and tilt your head forward slightly. It is in this position that we can best absorb, comprehend and retain. I think we can agree that if you sit up straight but tilt your chin up slightly, reading becomes more difficult. In order to chew, digest and absorb information completely, we must sit up straight, head tilted slightly forward so the head spiral is pointing upward. The same holds true if our aim is to circulate, digest and absorb what we eat.

In this position, sitting up straight with your head spiral facing upward, the food remains in your mouth as you chew—it doesn't slip down your throat—and you can circulate (chew) the food as many times as you wish—fifty times, a hundred times, five hundred times. In order to chew thoroughly and well, it's best to put down your utensils between each mouthful and place your hands in your lap. This increases your concentration and encourages thorough chewing.

Why do I place so much emphasis on chewing? Chewing strengthens digestion. If you chew your food well, you will develop your physical ability to digest and assimilate food.

Chewing and circulation

Chewing is a pump. It circulates all our body's energy and fluids, all blood, lymph, digestive, hormonal and cellular fluids. Each chew is like a pump circulating all our energy. Each chew is renewing our physical, emotional, mental and spiritual health. To digest food properly, the minimum count is thirty. To quiet the mind and develop thinking, the minimum is fifty. To refine ki (energy), the minimum is one hundred.

In Eastern philosophy, the body is made up of different systems working together and complementing each other. The digestive system and the brain form one of these systems. The digestive system is designed to digest solid and liquid food, the brain to digest vibrational food—food that takes the form of thoughts and images.

Chewing food—chewing ideas

Once, while I was living in Japan, I was invited to a restaurant that specialized in fugu, a treasured Japanese delicacy. Fugu is very expensive. It has a delicious and delicate taste but it is also highly poisonous. In fact, if it has not been properly prepared, it is usually fatal. Two days before I was scheduled to eat at this restaurant a famous sumo wrestler died of fugu poisoning, a fact which only served to increase my nervousness. But it would have been a terrible loss of face to turn down such an honored invitation so I went. I drank sake and ate fugu with my Japanese friends. None of them seemed unsettled by what had happened to the sumo wrestler but I wondered if this was to be my last meal. I tried to behave naturally even though I was frightened and eventually I managed to relax a bit. The fugu was delicious. To this day I don't know whether it was the taste and texture or the danger it posed that made it so interesting to eat.

Later, I told this story to a well-known Japanese macrobiotic teacher, Herman Aihara. He had a good laugh and then said, "A macrobiotic person can't be poisoned. His body won't accept the poison. It will immediately be thrown out of his body. You didn't have to worry."

Maybe, maybe not. But what I do believe is that we can be poisoned by ideas as readily as we can by food, perhaps more readily. If Eastern thinking is correct about the connection between the brain and the digestive system, then strengthening the digestive system is the easiest way to strengthen thinking ability. In other words, chewing your food and chewing your ideas amount to the same thing. If you chew your food well, you strengthen your ability to digest and assimilate ideas and thoughts. The action of chewing actually improves your thinking ability and your memory. A healthy mind can accept all ideas, chew them over and either absorb or dispel them. I call this conscious chewing. The concept is applicable to all forms of nourishment, physical, mental, emotional and spiritual.

Chewing and consciousness

It's important to be conscious of how you eat. Most people eat automatically. They give little or no thought to eating mindfully. Being relaxed before sitting down to eat will help you take the time to chew properly. Doing some stretching, a few yoga postures, or even some deep slow breathing before you start may help you to unwind.

A five to ten minute break between cooking and eating can make a big difference in your ability to enjoy your meal and to concentrate on chewing well. Cooking tends to be tightening and that may contribute to overeating and under-chewing.

You've probably not thought much about chewing. The fact is that most people chew very little. Changing old habits is tough so before you begin your new program of proper chewing observe the way you and other people chew. You'll be surprised at what you see and, with a bit of reflection, you'll soon realize that your body deserves better treatment.

Solid food should be chewed until it turns to liquid. Aim to chew each mouthful of food fifty times. Start slowly. For the first two weeks chew each mouthful twenty-five times. Work your way gradually to fifty or, if you have the will and the patience, to one hundred. Once you become accustomed to well-chewed food, you will feel uncomfortable if you eat too quickly.

The more you chew, the more aware you become of your own needs. People today tend to be constantly on the run with little or no time to reflect on what is important to them in their lives. Chewing well will help you break that pattern. It leads naturally to a calmer and more orderly life. By thinking about what's appropriate for you to do next, you will begin to use your time more efficiently and that, in turn, will help you accomplish more than you ever thought possible.

Everything in nature occurs in an alternating pattern—movement followed by rest—action followed by inaction. Ideally our lives should reflect this process. We might think we are wasting time if we stop to take care of ourselves and chew our food but, in reality, valuing our quiet time will make our active time more productive.

If you can take at least one or two of your three daily meals alone, you will have the ideal opportunity to concentrate on chewing well. Even if you can chew well at only one meal, you will notice an improvement in how you feel and think. If you can form the habit of chewing well at every meal, your health and your outlook on life will improve dramatically. You can chew well even when dining with others. Take advantage of those times when your companion is talking to do your chewing.

Chewing and digestion

Chewing well also releases the full power of saliva. Generally, saliva has a pH factor of 7.2, which means it is slightly alkaline. Saliva digests complex carbohydrates by breaking them down from complex to simple sugars. (That's why grains, beans and vegetables get sweeter the longer you chew them.) Chewing any food well prepares it to pass more smoothly and completely through the digestive system. Saliva can also neutralize imbalances in your food. Even if your diet is not well balanced, thorough chewing helps compensate for the imbalances.

When you chew well, your saliva mixes with the food and makes the food more alkaline, which means the food is better able to absorb the highly acidic secretions that are released in your stomach. If your blood is more alkaline, you will enjoy better health, stronger immunity and a greater resistance to illness.

Simple carbohydrates and refined foods are absorbed quickly into the blood stream, creating more acidic blood. Sugar and alcohol are simple carbohydrates. Many foods contain hidden sugar and sugar can be disguised in various ways on food labels. Most cakes, pastries, cookies and crackers contain sugar. Fruit is also a simple carbohydrate. Concentrated fruit juices are commonly used as sweeteners in many commercial and health food related products. These are all absorbed quickly and they all create acidic blood. Fructose, or fruit sugar, which is found in fruit and honey, can also raise blood cholesterol.

Other foods that are absorbed quickly include white rice, white bread, white pasta and potatoes. You can help neutralize their acidity by chewing thoroughly but it's best to avoid these foods altogether once your cravings are minimized.

The problem with these foods is that by the time they reach the stomach, they will have been absorbed in the mucous membranes and therefore will not pass through the duodenum. Foods that are absorbed before passing through the duodenum create more acidic blood. The duodenum has strong alkaline secretions that increase the alkalinity of our food before it passes into the small intestine for final digestion and absorption.

Opposites attract. Chewing alkalizes food. Then the alkaline food attracts stomach acids and the protein content is digested. Food turns alkaline again as it passes through the duodenum where fats are broken down. Your food is then ready for the next stage—final digestion and absorption in the small intestine. Only food that is absorbed through the small intestine creates healthy, alkaline blood. The final stage is water absorption and bowel formation in the colon or large intestine, where the waste products are then excreted.

When your blood is acidic, valuable minerals, especially calcium, are lost from bones, teeth, or muscles. These stored minerals are needed to create the buffer action that breaks down strong acid and turns it into weak acid on its way to being converted to carbon dioxide and water. Mineral loss dilutes the blood and weakens resistance to illness. It weakens the bones as well.

Acid blood weakens the kidneys, heart and lungs, all organs affected by excessive liquids. The kidneys must work harder to filter more blood and discharge more fluid which leads to a loss of valuable nutrients (minerals, B vitamins and vitamin C). The heart has to work harder to pump the increased blood volume. And the lungs must work harder also, in order to discharge the excess carbon dioxide and fluid. Think of the steam that emanates from our mouths when we exhale on a cold day. Think of how much more difficult it is to breathe easily when the weather is humid. Experiment. Try drinking a lot of fruit juice, beer, or soda before exercising. Check your heart and breathing rates and compare the readings with those taken when you drink fewer liquids.

As you can imagine, your health will be adversely affected by a loss of minerals. If you eat a steady diet of refined foods and white sugar, you will weaken your entire system and create a climate for the development of illness.

On the other hand, if you eat foods with healthful, nourishing complex carbohydrates and chew them well, you will enjoy the natural sweetness of good food that can be digested properly. Chewing regulates peristalsis, the automatic expansion and contraction of the muscles of the entire digestive system. Peristaltic movement is wavelike and forms a continuous pattern. Chewing stimulates peristalsis. The more you chew the more frequently the wavelike movement occurs and the more rapidly you move toward a state of balance.

The result is that elimination will return to normal and toxic conditions in the colon, conditions that could cause discomfort and disease, will be warded off. You will have reached the point at which the rhythm of your entire system flows in harmony with the rhythm of nature and the universe.

Thorough chewing makes the salivary glands produce enzymes that stimulate the release of parotid hormones. These hormones help the thymus gland create T cells, which bolster the immune system.

As I said earlier, chewing also acts as a pump that circulates the body's fluids and energy. Chewing actually activates the blood and other fluid circulation in the body as well as regulating energy flow. If you are feeling physically or emotionally blocked, chewing will help to disperse the stagnation that is causing those conditions. It activates the whole system and dispels negative energy.

Brighten up your day

After you have chewed thoroughly for a few days or longer, you will notice that you feel brighter and that you are thinking more clearly. This is also easy to test. Try chewing every mouthful of food, even soup and liquids, at least fifty times for four days. Notice the difference. Are you calmer? Is your thinking clearer? Is your energy brighter? If you feel adventurous, try another four days of chewing each mouthful of food at least one hundred times.

To make this a more useful test, it's best to count the number of chews per mouthful over the four-day period. Better chewing alone will strengthen your health but, as I said earlier, make sure that you are seated when you eat and not doing other things—not driving, watching TV or reading.

Relieving stress

Most people think they are wasting time when they take time for their meals. The busier and more stressed they are, the more they think they're wasting time. Nothing could be further from the truth. Consider this: the more you rush your meal, the more stressed you become. It's really quite simple. Traditionally there were three times during the day when we stopped what we were doing in order to return to balance, to re-nourish ourselves and readjust our direction. They were called meals—not lunch or dinner breaks—three times a day when we could stop and think, what am I doing, where am I going, what do I want to be doing? If we don't take time for meals we never develop the ability to ask or answer these questions and the result is that we lose our direction in life, we lose control over our lives. This is what we see happening today. People are more confused and disoriented than ever before. They never take the time to stop and think about the important things. Meals are purposeful in that they give us the opportunity for this kind of self-reflection. Meals are great stress relievers, provided they are at least twenty minutes long. You will gain time, not lose it, when you take time for your meals.

Highlights:

- Start by chewing each mouthful twenty to thirty times and gradually increase to fifty.

- To improve your health and calm your mind more quickly, chew each mouthful of food at least fifty times.

- Thorough chewing also helps you eat less and feel more satisfied.

- Chewing circulates your body's energy and all its fluids (blood, lymph, hormones, digestive, etc.).

- Put your utensils down after each mouthful. This will help you chew more thoroughly.

STOP EATING THREE HOURS BEFORE BEDTIME.

Your body cleans and repairs itself while you sleep. Your stomach needs to be empty for this process to be efficient. It takes, on average, about three hours for food to leave the stomach. Therefore, it's best to refrain from eating for three hours before retiring. My analogy is this: It's impossible to clean a room packed with people. If you want to clean a room thoroughly and efficiently, you have to empty it of people. If you want to clean your body, you have to empty it of food.

During the day while we're up and about, we receive the benefits of the sun's energy. Just the opposite occurs at night when we are nourished by celestial energy from the moon, stars, constellations and galaxy. Daytime is for activity, productivity and the spending of energy; nighttime is for rest, rejuvenation and the receiving of energy.

The body cannot perform the miraculous nocturnal task of rejuvenation unless the stomach is empty. Nor can we receive celestial energy at night unless we are empty inside. Food is condensed energy. When you eat, most of your food turns into energy in your body. If you go to sleep too soon after eating, your body will be too full of energy to do its nighttime work. Imagine a roomful of people and then imagine trying to clean, organize and rearrange that room. Difficult, wouldn't you say? But once the room is empty it's simple. Can you see from my analogy that your body is in a similar fix if it's not empty? When your stomach is too full, the body is so busy dealing with digestion it can't properly do its normal nighttime job. It's all too easy for the body to fall behind schedule when it can't discharge the toxins that accumulate in our cells and organs each day—which is exactly what happens when it's not allowed to repair itself each night.

> "To lengthen thy life, lessen thy meals."
>
> —Benjamin Franklin

Hypoglycemia

Here's another important point: When we eat, we secrete insulin in order to digest our food. If we eat before sleep, we go to sleep with too much insulin circulating in our bloodstream so that when morning comes we feel tired and sluggish and have a hard time getting up. This is one of the symptoms of hypoglycemia.

Let me tell you a little bit about hypoglycemia. The food we take before going to sleep is food that the body can't metabolize because it is in a prone position. This food goes to the liver for storage. The liver takes care of fat metabolism but it also has another important role. The liver neutralizes acidity and therefore helps keep our blood alkaline. When we eat before sleeping, we experience an increased build up of fat and cholesterol in our bloodstream which, in turn, promotes acidity. And acidic blood is a chief contributor to feelings of fatigue and stress. The excess, undigested food actually exhausts the body, which is unable to process and digest in a reclining position.

Among our vital organs, the liver, pancreas, kidneys and intestines are particularly over worked. Of course, many people feel they have to eat just in order to sleep. This is a symptom of hypoglycemia. What it means is that your blood sugar has fallen too low for you to fall asleep. Then the body demands that you eat in order to raise your blood sugar level, knowing that it will fall further while you sleep.

Even if what you eat at nine or ten at night is of good quality and healthful, you won't receive the best value from it. It may satisfy your appetite but without time to digest it properly you are effectively losing some of its benefits. Foods that are high in fiber and low in fat (i.e. complex carbohydrates), are digested more quickly and easily than animal and dairy foods. They contain less condensed energy and are easier for your body to process and, if you are up and about and active, their energy will disperse more quickly. But even the smallest amount of meat is so laden with condensed energy that it creates an even bigger burden on your body, so much of one that probably you would need more than a three hour wait before going to sleep.

> "A full belly makes a dull brain."
> —Benjamin Franklin

Cleaning your body and better sex

If you are recovering from an illness, you will benefit from allowing three to four hours of not eating before bedtime. Eating has a nourishing, expansive effect on the body. Cleaning or detoxifying is a process of taking out rather than taking in. Waiting more than three hours before bedtime enhances the body's ability to clean and repair itself during sleep. Experiment with the number of hours you allow yourself between the completion of your meal and your bedtime. When you allow more time, I am sure you will feel the difference the next day. For the record, the suggestion to stop eating three hours before bedtime means you should stop eating three hours before getting into bed or stretching out in a chair with your feet up to watch TV or to read. If your body is horizontal, you haven't complied with the suggestion. You will need to wait an additional three hours if you want to have the best digestion and the best sleep. If you reserve the bed exclusively for sleeping and sex, I'm sure you'll find both activities more rewarding.

Eating before sleep is a hard habit to break. At the same time, you need to realize that you can't have really good health unless you do break it. If you can't go to sleep without eating for three hours beforehand, the most likely cause is that you're not satisfied with the meals you took during the day. The only way to overcome this habit is to make the day's meals more satisfying. Pay particular attention to breakfast, followed by lunch. People who like to be very active and busy don't often sit down for a complete meal during the course of the day. They can't spare the time and they don't want to be slowed down by food. Often they will eat dinner at a very late hour. Whether they eat early or late, this type of person usually feels more relaxed after dinner and it is this overdue relaxation that stimulates late night hunger.

Not eating before sleep sounds easy but it's not. It may require some life style changes.

Highlights:

- To promote the best health, finish your evening meal by eight p.m. Let a full three hours pass before lying down. Stretching out in bed or even on a chaise lounge does not allow for good digestion.

- It takes about three hours for your stomach to empty after you finish eating.

- Your stomach must be empty for your body to clean, repair and recharge itself efficiently while you sleep.

- You will sleep more deeply, need fewer hours and awake more refreshed.

- Anything you eat before going to sleep—good food or bad—goes to the liver for storage and prevents your liver from getting a rest and repairing itself.

EAT IN AN ORDERLY MANNER.

Balance has a certain kind of order. You may think what I am about to propose is a very rigid way to eat. A number of older macrobiotic friends have told me just that. My answer is that I'm still here actively counseling and teaching macrobiotics and they aren't. So I'll stick with my way.

What is my way? Let's take dinner: You can start your meal with soup, followed by a grain and a few different side dishes and end it with dessert and/or a beverage, if you choose.

Two types of soup

There are two main types of soup: savory and sweet. Savory soups are well seasoned and mildly salty. Their purpose is to stimulate and activate digestion. Vegetable soup, shoyu soup and miso soup (vegetable soup seasoned with miso) are savory. Among the three, miso soup has the most ability to promote good digestion.

Sweet vegetable soups are pureed and have a mild, pleasantly sweet and creamy taste—squash soup, onion, cabbage, and leek soup and carrot soup are some examples. The purpose of sweet vegetable soup is to harmonize, balance and relax the digestive system.

Savory soup should be started at the beginning of the meal. Whether you finish it before going on to the rest of your meal or continue to consume it throughout the meal, as if it were a side dish, is up to you. There is actually more benefit in taking this type of soup throughout the meal. Sweet vegetable soup doesn't have the same ability to activate digestion but there's no harm in starting your meal with it. Since it lightens, relaxes and opens up the digestive system, we can enjoy it throughout the meal as well.

Miso soup is a wonderful way to start the day; however, some people who take miso soup for breakfast can't stop eating all day! It makes them excessively hungry. In those cases, I recommend against it. It's better to take it at lunch or dinnertime. But if you're comfortable with it in the morning and it doesn't cause you to overeat, just keep on with it.

Grain from beginning to end

Grain is eaten throughout the meal from beginning to end. Now let's talk about vegetable dishes which are interspersed with the grain. As I said earlier, balance has a certain kind of order. To achieve balance, it's best to follow that order. Take some grain, chew it thoroughly then move on to the vegetable side dishes. Start with the heavier, long cooked dishes and finish with the lighter, more quickly cooked ones.

Let's go through the order of a meal together. Start the meal with soup. Then take a mouthful of grain, chew it and swallow it. If you're having a bean (or bean product such as tofu or tempeh), take that next followed by another mouthful of grain. Then move on to a sea vegetable, such as hijiki or arame, if you're having one. Take a mouthful, chew that and swallow it. If you're not quite satisfied by one mouthful of sea vegetable, have another, have two or three if you wish. Take some grain and then go on to whatever other long cooked vegetable you may be having. Take another mouthful of grain and then return to the beans followed by the long cooked vegetable, then the grain and then move on to the more quickly cooked vegetable dishes, those that have been sauteed, steamed or blanched, for instance. My definition of a lightly or quickly cooked vegetable is this: the crunching sound you make while chewing a lightly cooked vegetable should be audible to the person sitting next to you. No crunch means the vegetable is overcooked. Remember to intersperse the grain with the other dishes. Grain is taken consistently throughout the meal. The salad (pressed salad before raw salad) is taken at the end of the meal. Dessert, if you choose to have one, and tea complete the meal.

A meal eaten in this manner has a wavelike pattern. Think of yourself sitting on the beach, watching the tide go out. The tide doesn't go out all at once, does it? No, it waves out. In other words, it goes out but comes back in a bit, out again but back in a bit, and so on. My point is that although the tide continues to come in, overall it's gradually moving out. In the same way, although grain is taken consistently from the beginning to the end of the meal, overall the meal is moving in a certain direction.

Just to avoid confusion let me say the following: Adults generally don't finish one dish before going on to the next but you can if that is your preference. Generally, most children eat through one dish at a time. They like everything to be as simple as possible. Often they don't like it if the different foods on their plates are even touching. If you wish to develop direct, simple, childlike thinking you can eat this way. If, however, you want to think more elaborately, then you should move back and forth, in a wavelike pattern. So you are constantly coming back while moving further and further out—like the tide.

Highlights:

- Orderly eating aids digestion and promotes clear thinking. It will leave you feeling more satisfied.

- If you are having soup, start the meal with it. You may finish your soup before going on to the rest of the meal or you may eat it throughout the meal.

- Eat grains from the beginning to the end of the meal.

- Gradually move from the heavier, well-cooked dishes to the lighter, more quickly cooked or raw dishes. Salads come last and are followed by dessert and tea.

- It is not necessary to finish one dish before moving on the next. The pattern is a wave like motion that resembles the tide as it goes out.

- Orderly eating leads to orderly thinking.

AVOID MIXING FOODS IN THE SAME MOUTHFUL.

Keep the foods on your plate distinct and separate, not touching. Imitate the child in this respect. To accomplish this you either have to take smaller portions or put the different foods in small individual dishes as the Japanese do. I don't like to put everything on my plate at once so I only take a couple of dishes at a time and then go back for the others. It often happens that my children finish the foods I like before I'm ready to refill my plate. It's no different when I'm at the Strengthening Health Institute's residential programs. The outcome is that I'm prevented from overeating! Everything is as it should be.

Why do I stress keeping the food on our plates from touching? Digestion is a mechanical process. For instance, if you mix two foods together in the same mouthful, digestive enzymes are going to attach to one food more than to the other. That's their nature. The process works like this: the mouth secretes saliva. Saliva is alkaline. Whichever food becomes more alkalized by the saliva will attract more stomach acid which, in turn, will attract more alkaline secretions in the duodenum when it arrives there.

That food will be well absorbed in the small intestine and equally so in the large intestine. But the other food will miss out completely. Different foods are digested differently.

If you cook two foods together, such as pressure-cooked rice and beans or stir-fried grain and vegetables, they can be eaten together. They have blended in the cooking process. They are no longer two distinct foods. But if you cook rice and beans separately, eat them separately. Don't put the beans on your rice. There are exceptions. If you cook two dishes separately but mix them together while they're still hot, the residual heat will cause them to blend. In effect, they become one dish. If you want to make a grain and vegetable salad using leftover rice, reheat the rice then add the vegetables, whether they are raw or previously cooked or freshly cooked. The heat from the rice will allow the ingredients to blend and become digestible. You can let the dish cool down to room temperature before eating it if that is your preference. It is still one dish. Energetically this is entirely different from mixing distinct foods together on your plate or in your mouth. It's crucial not to mix different foods in the same mouthful. Foods cooked separately should be chewed separately.

As I've already mentioned, children don't like different foods to touch on their plates and, in general, they like simple dishes. But, under some circumstances they do mix everything together. When? When they don't like what they are eating and just want to get it down. When are adults most likely to mix foods together, when they have a healthy appetite and are full of energy or when their appetite is sluggish and they feel tired?

Here's another question. What stimulates your mind more, eating distinct dishes or eating those that have been mixed together on the plate? The answer, of course, is eating each dish individually. If you eat this way, you will see an improvement in both your digestion and your ability to think.

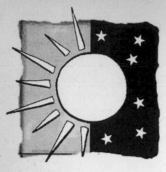

STEP 2

SET YOUR
DAILY SCHEDULE

RISE EARLY AND SLEEP BEFORE MIDNIGHT.

Rise early to be more active and discharge more toxins. The time at which you get out of bed in the morning—not your waking time—is what sets the tone for your day. If you want to be more active and productive, get out of bed by seven a.m. at the latest. If you leave your bed at nine or even worse, at eleven a.m., there's a sense in which you might as well not bother to leave it at all.

Think about this: the sun rises with a burst of energy that cleans and refreshes everything on earth. When you get out of bed around the time of sunrise, you can take full advantage of this burst of energy. It is at this time that your body has the greatest capacity to discharge excess, to clean and refresh itself. Within an hour or two after sunrise, the sun's movement starts to slow down. By nine a.m. it has slowed down considerably. Let's take a look at exactly what happens when you get up late, as many people do on Sundays. You have a late breakfast—referred to as brunch—usually sometime between ten and noon, a time when we're meant to be active. Now if we eat when we're meant to be active, we get very sluggish. We lie around for the rest of the day, reading the paper, dragging from one thing to another. The effect on us is the same as if we had overeaten, isn't it? Why should this be the case? The answer is that we don't have the ability to digest or process the sun's energy when we're in a horizontal position. The sun's energy is very coarse. We absorb it through the head spiral located toward the back part of the top of the head and for this to occur we have to be upright.

If you eat a big meal during the day, afterwards you feel sluggish, you can't think clearly. Even if you take an afternoon nap in a darkened room, you still feel sluggish when you awake. You don't have to be directly exposed to the sun's rays for this to happen. If we are horizontal when the sun is up, we don't have the ability to process the sun's energy. The immune system is effectively deactivated and the overall effect on us is the same as that of overeating.

It's just as important for our health to be asleep before midnight as it is to rise with the sun. During the night we receive very subtle energy from the celestial world, the moon, stars and planets. As we sleep, we are nourished by this celestial influence. We have to be horizontal for this energy to be most effectively absorbed. Our deepest sleep occurs between one a.m. and three a.m. Celestial vibrations are strongest between midnight and four a.m., at the time when the most stars are visible in the sky, the greatest number being visible at about two a.m. It takes an hour or two to fall into the deepest sleep, so we need to be asleep by eleven p.m. to receive the optimal celestial influence and, therefore, the best results for our health. If this is difficult, given the demands of modern society, try to be in bed by midnight.

> "Early to bed and early to rise, makes a man healthy, wealthy and wise."
>
> *—Benjamin Franklin*

I have read that we need a certain number of hours of sleep and if we don't get them we have to "catch up." If you think about this, it doesn't make much sense. How well or poorly we sleep is determined by our diet and activity during the day. If we eat too much or too little, it's hard to sleep. The same holds true for activity. If we sit around all day, we probably will not sleep well. When we work too hard and exhaust ourselves, sleep often does not come easily. The amount of sleep we need is determined by how long it takes our body to clean, repair and recharge itself. The better our health, the less time we need for the cycle of cleaning, repairing and recharging. Most people find that they need considerably less sleep within a couple of weeks of adopting the Strengthening Health recommendations. If our diet and activity are not in balance every day, we won't sleep well at night and, if we don't sleep well at night, our body won't be able to clean, repair and re-energize its organs and nervous system. On the other hand, if our diet and activity are in balance, the sleeping process becomes very efficient, takes less time to achieve and gives us deeper sleep. The result is that we feel rested and refreshed with fewer hours of sleep.

If we are in good health, either a rich, elaborate meal or a light simple one will satisfy us and provide good energy. The same principle applies to the subject of sleep. The average person in good health requires five to seven hours of sleep. If we get a little less than that, we will still feel fine and, if we choose to sleep a bit longer, perhaps on the weekend, we'll also feel fine. The bottom line is that when we are in good health, we can be flexible about how much we eat and the amount of sleep we need.

Let's consider the quality of sleep. Deep sleep, undisturbed by dreams, is the most refreshing. If you spend the night dreaming, the mind does not have the opportunity to relax and recharge. If you follow the Strengthening Health suggestions accurately, you will not experience confusing or disturbing dreams and you will awaken with the will and the energy to pursue what you want out of life— to pursue your real dreams.

Everyone is concerned with getting a good night's sleep. If you live in proper rhythm with nature, eat at regular scheduled intervals, chew your food well and allow enough time before bed for digestion, you will have no problem with sleep.

Highlights:

- Your rising time regulates your energy and activity for the day. Aren't you less productive if you get up late?

- Rise by seven a.m. to be more active and discharge more toxins. Your body has the greatest ability to discharge excess early in the morning.

- Be asleep before midnight to sleep more deeply, awake more refreshed and be physically stronger.

- Your body can clean and repair itself more efficiently when you are asleep before midnight.

KEEP YOUR MEALTIMES REGULAR.

Regular meals regulate all of your body's cycles—physical, emotional and mental. They make your energy and life more stable. It's important to take your meals at approximately the same time every day. This adjustment alone will greatly improve your health. As easy as this step may sound, the reality is that it takes time and discipline to rethink this aspect of your life. As the world has gotten more complicated, the manner in which we take our most important nourishment is often ignored.

Think about your mealtimes during the past week. Were you able to sit down to your meals at approximately the same time each day? Did you even take the time to sit down when eating breakfast or lunch? If your answer is no, you aren't alone. Most people don't realize the importance of maintaining a regular meal schedule and don't think they are undermining their health by not eating at regular times. But their health is surely suffering.

Even if you still eat meat and potatoes every day, just doing it at regular intervals will let you benefit from your food far more than if you eat these same foods in a disorderly manner. The body responds positively to a set schedule and is very grateful when it is allowed to align itself with nature—so grateful that it will reward you abundantly with better mental and physical health. This is because the time at which we eat determines how well we digest our food.

When do we have the most active digestion? To answer this question I have to ask another. Actually, it's a trick question. Should we eat our meals when we're hungry or should we eat at regular specified times? The answer is that if we eat regular meals and if we don't overeat, then we will be hungry at mealtimes. Why should this be so?

Aligning with Nature

Mealtimes are not arbitrary. They are part of the natural cycle of life. Everything in life is governed by the sun's movement, whether throughout the day or throughout the year. The sun has three extreme positions—sunrise, sunset and the high point in the sky, noon. The extreme angles of the sun indicate what we call mealtimes. The time in between these angles is for activity.

Most people are active in the morning and in the spring, less active in the middle of the night or in the dead of winter. Breathing is more active in the daytime and in the summer and is quieter at night and in the winter.

What breakfast really encourages is rising and separating energy. In the morning, we rise and separate from our families and/or our homes; we all go off in different directions—we separate and enter the larger world. This is the energetic effect of sunrise. We get up, wash, brush our teeth, have breakfast or not and then leave the house for work, for school, for errands, etc. The usual pattern is one of separating from family and home.

Lunch is a time for either activity or stagnation, depending on when and what we eat. Lunch can give us uplifting, active energy or sinking, stagnating energy. If we want to be active after lunch, we should eat early and the meal should be simple and complete. People who are physically active generally eat a light early lunch. In Spain, lunch is an elaborate meal that is served very late. Since no one can stay awake after such a large and late meal, lunch is quite naturally followed by a long siesta.

Dinner is a time for returning home, a time to gather and unify. Until recently, at least, families ate dinner together, perhaps talking, perhaps arguing but in any event sharing the events and experiences of the day. Family members communicated, unified and aligned as a family. This alignment and reunification also follows a natural pattern or tendency.

The nature of energy or of vibrations, as I've mentioned before, is such that vibrations try to align. In other words, they try to become similar in their quality, speed and direction of movement. Think of a moving merry-go-round. If you want to step on smoothly, you have to be moving in the same direction and at the same speed as the merry-go-round itself. If you are moving faster or slower, your boarding will be jerky because the two different energies are not aligning properly. And, furthermore, should you approach a merry-go-round from the direction opposite to its movement, you will be thrown off even as you attempt to climb on.

Another example of the alignment of energy is this one: Imagine a meeting room filled with vegans who have just finished dinner. Generally, vegans have more peaceful energy because they eat a grain and vegetable based diet without meat or dairy products. Let's say they drink herbal tea at the end of their meal and as a result are even calmer and more peaceful than usual. In our scenario, these vegans are discussing various types of meditation when someone new enters the room, momentarily disrupting the conversation. Let's say that the newcomer has just left the local sports bar where he has eaten a dinner of fried chicken washed down with a few beers. The atmosphere in the bar was heated because the local hockey team was losing. You can appreciate that this person's energy would be very strong, perhaps even jarring compared with the energy of the vegans. The group would no doubt lose its focus and wonder who this guy was and why he was there. Do you see the problem? The newcomer's energy is just too different for it to align quickly with the energy of the others. Either the newcomer or the vegans will feel uncomfortable. Only as time passes will their energy even start to align.

When members of a family come together on a daily basis, they build understanding and communication. So long as this they do this, the family will function harmoniously. Each of us goes out every day and encounters many different influences and experiences. We eat different foods, talk to different people, engage in different activities, all of which alter our condition and thinking. We align with individuals outside the family through common or similar points and qualities. This is not a threat to the family but an asset—as long as we continue to take our evening meal together. Understanding and communication develop as we talk and eat together. We can go out again after dinner, if we choose. As long as the unification process, the aligning process continues at the evening meal, the family's stability and balance will develop and be maintained.

Breakfast, Lunch and Dinner

Now that we know that meals are meant to align us with nature's energy let's talk specifically about breakfast, lunch and dinner. As I said earlier, breakfast should give us rising and separating energy so that we can be in harmony with the natural world. The sun rises, the dew evaporates, flowers open. Breakfast the world over has one ingredient in common and that is liquid. When, for instance, we boil water for tea or coffee, the boiling water evaporates, creating rising and separating energy. Whether breakfast consists of cold cereal with milk, porridge (the difference between a macrobiotic person's breakfast grain and dinner grain is simply the amount of liquid used), miso soup, orange juice, coffee, tea or simply a glass of water, liquid is the common ingredient. It is what we need to rise and separate. A breakfast consisting of bacon, eggs and dry toast makes for a difficult day. The food is too dry to create active, separating energy. If we want to get moving, we would have to spread some jam on our toast and have a glass of juice or a cup of coffee. It's the liquid that enables us to be active in the morning. If breakfast is too dry, we're not able to align with nature's rising and separating energy. On the other hand, we can still function perfectly well if we take just liquid for breakfast.

Breakfast time is also the time to separate from home. If you work at home and don't leave the house before you settle down, if you go from your bed to your office or your studio, perhaps by way of the bathroom and kitchen, I think you'll find that after a while you lose your creativity and your drive. There is simply no polarity. If you work at home, my suggestion is that you go out and do something, then return. Have a cup of tea, buy a newspaper or just take a walk around the block. Unless you have some degree of separation after breakfast, you'll find that you become tired and stale as the morning wears on.

Dinner is a different matter. Dinner should be more substantial—longer cooked and not too watery—too much liquid can interfere with sleep. If at dinner we drink too much beer, wine, apple juice, soda, coffee or tea—the common point being liquid—we can't sleep. (Sugar changes to water in the body, which means we have to watch our intake of simple carbohydrates also.) Dinner should give us settling down and gathering energy since it coincides with the setting of the sun. Dinner is the most suitable meal at which to have a protein.

Imagine your day if you swapped breakfast and dinner. You could no longer align with nature's energy. Mealtimes are not arbitrary, as I said earlier. The meal is our way of aligning with nature's energy no matter where we are—even if we live in the middle of Manhattan in a high-rise made of materials that carry an incredible electromagnetic charge, a place where we couldn't be more isolated from nature. If we have regular meals that consist of appropriate ingredients for the time of day, we will be able to align with nature's energy. By contrast, if we live in the most pristine setting and eat chaotically, we may be surrounded by nature but we are not aligning with it. Meals create our connection to nature. I think of the meal as an anchor that creates stability in our lives, no different from the anchor that keeps a ship from drifting into dangerous waters.

Lunch. Around lunchtime, the sun climbs to its highest point in the sky and appears to hang there motionless for a while before it begins its descent. There are two sorts of energy to choose from at lunchtime, one is active energy, the other is more stagnant. If you want to be active and productive in the afternoon, you would be wise to eat while the sun is still rising. If you wait to eat until it's hanging out at its high point, your energy for the afternoon will be more stagnant.

If we want to be active in the afternoon, at what time should we begin lunch? To answer this question, let's go back to the example I gave earlier. Think about the after-lunch siesta for which Spain is famous. When is lunch eaten in Spain? Usually, from two to four p.m. At twelve, should they even be open, the restaurants are empty. Portugal and Spain are next door to one another but Portugal has no siesta. In Portugal, lunch is eaten either from twelve to one p.m., or from one to two p.m. During the tourist season you can distinguish the Spanish from the Portuguese simply by the times they choose to eat. The Portuguese are leaving the restaurants as the Spaniards are entering. The different dining habits of these two cultures are emblematic of their different lifestyles. Nevertheless, in spite of the late hours at which they dine, Spaniards still rise with the sun and therefore enjoy long and productive mornings.

So, if you want to be active in the afternoon, finish lunch by two p.m. at the latest—one p.m. would be even better. The later you start lunch, the less you can accomplish afterwards. It's as simple as that. Remember that when you eat you are aligning with the sun's energy. Try this test. Eat similar lunch food every day for four weeks, but for the first two weeks start lunch at twelve p.m. For the following two weeks, start it at two p.m. You will certainly notice a difference. It's common knowledge that the best way to insure being useless in the afternoon is to eat a late, rich lunch.

Lunch should be simple yet complete and satisfying. Think of foods that allow you to remain physically and mentally active. The test is whether or not you can work, think and be productive after eating them. Here are a few possibilities using grains or grain products and quickly cooked vegetables: vegetable sushi rolls (brown rice and vegetables wrapped in toasted nori seaweed), rice balls, fried rice, fried noodles or noodles in broth and quick steamed vegetables or vegetable sautés. What qualifies as a simple and complete meal in our part of the world? The sandwich does. Sandwiches are simple and quick and can be complete and healthy depending on what's in them. Tofu, hummus or any vegetable-type spread served on steamed and unyeasted sourdough bread is an example of a nourishing sandwich. You can complement the sandwich with a bowl of vegetable soup and a vegetable side dish, a salad, for instance. Not so long ago, a lunch consisting of a bowl of soup, a sandwich and a pickle was a fairly typical meal.

Mealtimes

Should the main meal of the day be served at midday or at sunset? Well, there's a good argument for both. Agrarian societies took their main meal at noon and ate lightly in the evening. The advent of the Industrial Age changed that because a simple meal fit in better with the workday. Both will produce good health; choose what suits your lifestyle.

Try not to skip any meals. How much you eat is up to you; what is significant is the regularity. If you cannot make every meal regular, the most important one is your main meal of the day. Having a regular dinner, the gathering, unifying meal, provides the most benefit. When I say a meal should be served at the same time every day, I mean it. A fifteen-minute variation in the schedule is acceptable. Thirty minutes is pushing it. Remember that mealtimes regulate all your body's cycles so the timing is important for your health.

Your blood-sugar level is one function that follows the sun's movement, as do your activity and energy levels. Digestion, bowel movements, all of your physical and mental cycles—they, too, follow the sun's movement. So if you want regular digestion, regular bowel movements, regular menstruation, regular blood sugar levels and more balanced emotions, sit down to regular meals.

When I lived in Portugal, I spent a lot of time in the company of old friends who had been living there for a number of years. We shared many meals together. In some ways, they were more careful about what they ate than I was. Yet that family— both parents and children—did not enjoy good health. I believe there was a single reason. Even though they ate good quality food, they never sat down to regular meals. They ate when they were hungry and often they ate standing up.

Nothing has a stronger effect on regulating the body's cycles than regular meals. And nothing has a more disruptive effect than skipping meals, eating chaotically, or eating erratically.

The starting times for our three regular meals are as follows: Breakfast, five to seven a.m. Lunch, eleven a.m. to one p.m. Dinner, five to seven p.m. The time at which we eat determines how well or poorly we digest our food. The above are the times at which we have the most active digestion, the times at which we can digest our food most thoroughly. The principle behind this applies to sleep as well. Let's say you need five hours sleep a night. Which schedule will give you more energy: Sleeping from eleven p.m. to four a.m., or sleeping from four to nine a.m.? Clearly you are much better off sleeping from eleven p.m. to four a.m., rising when the sun rises, to take full advantage of the sun's energy.

Highlights:

- Regular meals regulate all your body's cycles, physical, emotional and mental.

- You will have better energy and digestion, more regular moods and clearer thinking.

- The time you start your meal regulates your metabolism. Start your meals earlier to be more active and productive. Breakfast: five to seven a.m. (eight a.m., at the latest). Lunch: eleven a.m. to one p.m. Dinner: five to seven p.m.

- Your health will improve more quickly and be more stable.

- Eat your meals at the same time everyday.

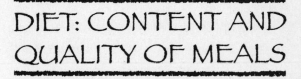

DIET: CONTENT AND QUALITY OF MEALS

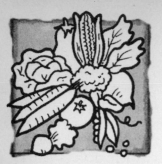

STEP 3

EAT TWO OR THREE BALANCED MEALS EVERYDAY

Grain and vegetable dishes together at the same meal provide the most complete and balanced nutrition.

> "A meal without a grain is just a snack."
>
> —*Michio Kushi*

PLAN EVERY MEAL AROUND COOKED GRAINS AND GRAIN PRODUCTS.

We have reached the end of a long dietary experiment. The concept of the pyramid comprised of the four basic food groups–animal products, dairy products, starches and fruits vegetables—was introduced by the Harvard Medical School in 1945. It is the model that many of us grew up with. Though it took more than fifty years, these government guidelines have finally been revised. The current recommendations strongly resemble the standard macrobiotic diet.

Of course, the government doesn't call it the standard macrobiotic diet even though grains and vegetables now occupy the base of the pyramid and constitute the highest percentage of the overall recommended diet. This indicates that there is certainly a new awareness of healthful nutrition. The government is, at last, trying to lead us in the right direction.

Cereal Grain

There is one major problem, however. Hardly anyone today knows what a cereal grain is. (Cereal grain was the traditional name for all grains.) If you ask people whether they eat cereal grains, the likely answer will be yes. That's because most of us think that dry breakfast cereals such as Cheerios, Rice Krispies and Corn Flakes are cereal grains. They are not. Most breakfast cereals are made with refined grain that is largely devoid of balanced nutrition. And, with few exceptions, breakfast cereals are loaded with sugar. To avoid confusion, I use the word 'grain' to mean cereal grain.

Although grain and grain products have nourished, sustained and developed the world's great civilizations for thousands of years, the average person is not quite sure what a grain really is. Traditionally, the Orient, Middle East, Africa, eastern and western Europe and the Americas all had grain-based diets. So let's talk about grains. Basically a grain is made up of three parts:

- Bran, the outer layer of the kernel, the part that protects the grain from oxidation. It contains protein, minerals, and vitamins.

- Germ, the heart of the life-giving part, contains oil and vitamins. It is actually the seed of the grain.

- Endosperm, the starchy bulk or center of the grain, is mostly carbohydrate. It is the fruit of the grain, the food the seed uses to grow.

A single grain contains the beginning and the end of all plant food since it merges the seed and the fruit into one. Grains and grain products are either "whole" or "refined." A grain is whole when all three of those parts are undisturbed and complete. A grain is refined when part or all of the bran or germ has been removed. The more of the bran and germ that is removed, the more refined the grain is. The more refined the grain, the more out of balance it is and the less nutritional value it has. Rice, wheat and corn are the principal grains grown for human consumption. Rice is used by more than half of the world's population and is seen most widely in one of two types—brown rice and white rice.

Brown rice is whole grain rice, with only the hull removed and it can be bought in any of three forms—short, medium, or long grain. Short and medium grain rice is more natural to temperate climates; long grain rice is preferable in hotter climates. Short grain rice contains more of a protein substance called gluten and when cooked it is somewhat stickier than long grain rice. Brown rice is the world's most balanced food and is extremely high in nutritional value. It should be eaten every day. Brown rice combines deliciously with all other foods, even foods that are not part of the macrobiotic diet. Amazingly, whatever is cooked in the same pot with brown rice will be thoroughly cooked in the same amount of time it takes to cook the rice.

White rice has had its hull, bran and germ removed so it does not begin to compare nutritionally with brown rice. You would have to eat seven times as much white rice as brown to ingest the same nutrients!

Referring to a familiar, everyday food such as rice as a "grain" seems to confuse people. Virtually everyone has eaten lots of rice over the years but probably without ever thinking of it as a grain. Rice is readily available and simple to cook and it's important that you make it a staple of your daily diet.

Another excellent way to ensure that your meal revolves around a grain is to eat pasta or noodles as your main food. I have yet to meet anyone who doesn't like pasta. I am referring, of course, to good quality pasta or noodles, not to those that contain ingredients such as eggs or sugar that are detrimental to health. Later in the book you will find a list of other grains, some of which are probably unfamiliar to you. It's best to start by eating brown rice and to develop the habit of making grains the focus of your meal.

When you are ready, visit the natural food section of your local supermarket or health food store and check out the grains. Incorporate those you are already familiar with into your diet. If they are already part of your diet, use them more regularly as the centerpiece of your meals. My suggestion is that you plan every meal around cooked grains and grain products. Then complete and balance every meal with one to two vegetable dishes. Activate and harmonize your digestion with a bowl of vegetable soup at one or two meals. And always buy the highest quality organically grown, unrefined and naturally processed foods you can find.

Grains and vegetables at every meal

Just as we use our meal times and rising and sleeping times to align externally with nature's cycles so we use the meal itself to align internally with our own biological cycles. Ongoing alignment with both cycles creates a powerful environment for the development of spiritual, emotional and physical health. We cannot create this important biological alignment without first defining what we mean by the word 'meal.' A meal consists of a grain or grain product and at least one separate vegetable dish. Even if the grain or grain product has many vegetables in it, such as stir-fried noodles and vegetables, it is classified as a grain dish. This being the case, we are still missing a separate vegetable dish. When we add the vegetable dish, we have a meal. What I'm saying is this: Your vegetable dish needs to be a separate dish, not vegetables cooked in or with something else, for example, in soup or in grains or grain products. Any vegetable cooked with grain becomes part of the grain dish. Any vegetable cooked in soup becomes part of the soup itself. To be annoyingly clear about this: The essence of a meal is a grain or grain product and at least one separate, stand alone vegetable dish.

"Tell me what you eat, and I will tell you what you are."

—Anthelme Brillat-Savarin

Principal foods

The term "principal food" refers to the food that is the centerpiece or core of the meal. In the modern American diet, protein in the form of meat or poultry or fish has been the most common principal food. In today's world, when a meal is planned the first decision to make is what protein to serve. The rest of the meal evolves from this starting point. Most of the world's long standing cultures, however, planned their meals around the grain dish and this is the format we use. The first question to ask is: "What grain or grain product will be the centerpiece of my meal?" We might choose brown rice, barley, noodles, good quality bread, polenta or cracked wheat, etc. The choice of grain is the center point around which the rest of the meal—which should include vegetables and other supplemental foods—should be planned.

Basic four

It's important to understand why grain was displaced as the world's principal food. Let's take a closer look at the 1945 Harvard Medical School guidelines and their four recommended food groups—animal food, dairy products, starches and fruits/vegetables. In the Harvard model, grains and vegetables, which in the past had been principal foods, became supplemental ones while animal and dairy foods, which previously had been supplemental foods, became principal foods—in a complete reversal of the natural order. After a time, people began to think of animal and dairy foods as indispensable to health. This notion was coupled with an idea in favor at the time: In order to form complete proteins, human beings needed a certain number of essential amino acids in their diet and these essential amino acids could be found only in animal and dairy foods.

As was later proved, these assumptions were completely inaccurate. All food has protein. We can get all of the essential amino acids from a combination of whole grains, beans and vegetables. We can include soy products such as tofu and tempeh to increase our protein intake. White-meat fish can be used as a further protein supplement. As we have learned to our detriment, it's a bad idea to overemphasize protein. Many modern diseases are the result of excessive protein intake.

The theory connecting animal foods and amino acids was promoted by the medical community, the news media and by the public school system. Consequently, millions of us learned at an early age that animal food was vital to our health. I think of this premise as a modern-day fallacy or a modern-day superstition.

Today we are hearing a different story. The new recommendations urge us to consume more grains and vegetables and fruits and to reduce or eliminate animal, dairy and other fatty foods from our diet. Sadly, most of us don't know what natural foods, such as grains and vegetables, are. We have no idea of the variety that awaits us. Mention vegetables and most people think of potatoes, lettuce, possibly frozen peas or carrots and, maybe, string beans. I have met children who think that carrots grow in little cubes. This is not an unreasonable assumption, if the only carrots you are familiar with come in a can.

The point is that natural foods, such as grains and vegetables, which all bestow health benefits have been out of the mainstream American diet for such a long time that they are now considered weird. If you mention the word rutabaga or parsnip, most people don't know if you're talking about a vegetable or a dance craze. I recently heard of a family in which the children actually used the word rutabaga to taunt and insult each other! We have gotten so far away from wholesome food that we as a nation need reeducation. Paradoxically, although we live in a high tech world that requires us to master very complicated material, for many of us the thought of having to acquire the simplest, most basic knowledge—how to improve our health through healthful eating—is overwhelming.

Cooking classes are the best starting place for your reeducation. Check the bulletin board of your natural food store for information on cooking classes, lectures or seminars on natural diet and life style. While you are there, pick up a cookbook or two. Cookbooks are good for ideas and inspiration once you have an understanding and image of healthy cooking and eating.

In the beginning stages, cooking can be learned only through personal experience. This is true of any style of cooking. To learn how to make a dish, we need to know three things—how the dish should look, how it should taste and how it should smell. We cook from an image and these factors form the basis of the image of whatever we are making. Once we have an image we can reproduce the dish. If, when eating out, I come across a dish I particularly like, I often replicate it at home—with slightly different ingredients, if necessary—but the point is, I always work from an image to create a new and healthy addition to my family's diet. In the past, people cooked using their intuition rather than cookbooks but many years of eating foods that do not properly nourish the brain or the spirit have hampered our intuition.

Moses in the Desert

Let's look at the biblical story of Exodus to better understand how natural foods disappeared from modern life. Moses took the Jewish people out of Egypt to deliver them from slavery into freedom. He wanted the Jews to build a new life free of the old enslaving concepts. However, the elders preferred what they knew to the possible dangers of the unknown. To fulfill his dream, Moses elected to have his people wander in the desert for forty years until the older generation died off. By then the young had grasped the idea of living in freedom. We have taken a more than fifty year long sojourn in the desert, journeying from a better way of eating to something far worse. During this time period, two important ideas were promoted.

The first was that science was somehow superior to nature, a corrective, in a manner of speaking. One significant myth was the notion that cow's milk or infant formula was healthier for babies than mother's milk. I was part of that experiment. My mother didn't nurse me. She fed me commercial baby formula followed by cow's milk. When I was in my twenties and learned about the physiological and psychological benefits of nursing for both mother and child, I asked her why she hadn't nursed me. She answered simply that at the time doctors thought bottle-feeding was superior. Now we know that nursing develops children's immunity, general health and thinking ability. It also helps children feel more secure emotionally and promotes a deeper bond between mother and child than bottle-feeding.

The second significant idea was that a diet based on animal and dairy foods was superior to one based on grains and vegetables. When the generation that had grown up with regular family meals died off, as in the story of Moses, the more natural way of eating, based on grains and vegetables, died with it.

Fast foods were introduced in the fifties. By the end of the sixties, people believed that eating when convenient was natural, that fast foods—hamburger, pizza, French fries and Coke—constituted a healthful diet; that processed breakfast cereals were grains and that white bread was a better choice than whole wheat or rye bread.

Over time, food technology became more and more sophisticated. Processed, frozen, canned, instant, microwave and chemically enhanced foods were introduced and popularized through massive advertising campaigns. They were heavily promoted even though they lacked the balanced and complete nutrition of natural, unprocessed foods.

There was a time when almost everyone started the day with a bowl of oatmeal, barley, Wheatena, Cream of Wheat or corn grits. Compare that practice with today's choice of bacon and eggs with white toast, bagels with cream cheese, or coffee with doughnuts and/or muffins. People also ate whole grain, unprocessed bread—whole wheat and rye breads that were freshly baked and chemical free. Until 1949, whole grain wheat bread was available commercially. Now commercial whole wheat bread is usually so refined that it is little more than glorified white bread. Pasta products and grains used to be of a much higher quality as well. Many people ate beans and a variety of seasonal fresh vegetables. Vegetable soup was considered essential daily fare. Yes, people did consume some animal and dairy food but usually in small portions and balanced by all the fresh, natural food in their diets. Even common snacks that people once enjoyed, such as seeds, nuts and dried fruits, have been more or less forgotten. And, in many parts of the country, anyone advocating healthy food choices is thought to be promoting some foreign diet.

A Great Way to Eat Food

"Macrobiotics is a great way to eat food." This is the answer given by my son, Joe, to the question, "What is macrobiotics?" I like the simplicity of his statement. It captures the feeling I have every time I sit down to eat. Once you are eating grains and vegetables on a regular basis you will be able to understand what Joe meant by his remark. At first, you will begin to feel better and to look younger and brighter. Your thinking and reasoning abilities will become keener. After a short while, you will notice that your taste buds have changed. When this happens, and it will happen quickly, you will stop craving food that is detrimental to your health. The body has its own wisdom and you will naturally crave healthier food. Hard as it is to believe, sooner or later, bacon and eggs will seem foreign to you!

I want to be clear about this: Americans must change their ideas about the meaning of complete nutrition. The modern practice of eating a lot of protein, especially animal protein, leads to serious illness. There is a real crisis in the health-care industry because health insurance companies cannot keep up with the huge numbers of people needing medical help and hospitalization. If you accept the concept that we are what we eat and that food can either make us sick or keep us well, then you must conclude that both as a nation and as individuals, we have been making the worst possible food choices for a very long time.

Grains and Vegetables

If we want good health, it is crucial that we return to a diet based on unrefined foods and complex carbohydrates. A grain or grain product and at least one vegetable dish should be eaten at every meal—including breakfast. This may take some getting used to but after a while if you aren't able to have a vegetable as part of your breakfast you will really miss having it. Vegetables complete cereal grains nutritionally and they will help you to feel more satisfied with your meals. Try to use a variety of cooking styles and a variety of vegetables because the more you vary both, the better your health will become. Green leafy vegetables, broccoli and cabbage are all excellent sources of calcium and vitamin C and they contain a surprising amount of protein.

Most of my children do not like "protein dishes." Some will eat beans occasionally, most like tofu but not tempeh and only a few of them like seitan (a wheat gluten product). Most of them do like fish but we serve fish only a few times a month. In spite of this, they are mostly in the top fifty percent of their grade for height and weight. Where does their protein for growth come from? The only possibility is the combination of grains and vegetables. Fruit, oil and grain based sweets are also a regular part of their diet and I am sure that these foods contribute to their growth as well.

Highlights:

- Grains and/or grain products are the centerpiece of a meal.

- Choose your grain first when planning a meal.

- Soft cooked grains such as oatmeal or soft rice are best for breakfast.

- Eat brown rice everyday.

- Grains have the ideal balance of minerals, proteins and carbohydrates that our body needs for balance and proper nourishment.

- You do not need to worry about the overall proportion of grains. Just eat a comfortable, satisfying amount.

COMPLETE AND BALANCE EVERY MEAL WITH ONE TO TWO VEGETABLE DISHES.

A Matter of Balance

What do we mean by balance? In order to feel satisfied, our bodies require a certain proportion of basic nutrients. We need approximately seven times more protein than minerals. This one-to-seven ratio represents a balance or an averaging of the numbers between one and ten and is not arbitrary. It derives from the workings of the natural environment. The rotation of the earth on its axis creates a powerful energy that we call earth's force—energy that is released upwards from the center of the earth. The movement of the universe also creates a powerful energy—energy that flows downwards toward the center of the earth and that we call heaven's force. Heaven's force is seven times greater than earth's force. This is why, in order to escape the earth's atmosphere and move into outer space, a rocket needs seven thousand pounds of thrust.

Around the world and down the centuries, definitions of balance and beauty have been based on this one-to-seven ratio. For example, classical Greek statues of the fourth century B.C., the Golden Age of Greece, have heads that are approximately one-seventh the size of their bodies. That which is aesthetically beautiful and pleasing to the human eye is not arbitrary either. Rather it is based on our innate sense of balance, a sense that comes directly from nature.

Many things conform to the one-to-seven ratio, including the ratio of nutrients necessary to maintain human health and well being. For example, if you eat a hard-boiled egg (concentrated protein), you will undoubtedly want to sprinkle some salt (minerals) on it. Salt improves the taste of eggs and makes them more digestible. Tofu needs soy sauce to make it tastier and easier to digest. The human body requires seven times as much carbohydrate as protein. If we eat meat, we quite naturally crave potatoes or beer or sugar—some type of carbohydrate—to balance the meat and make it digestible.

Grain is the only food that conforms to these ideal proportions. Grain contains about seven times as much protein as minerals and seven times as much carbohydrate as protein. Meat contains no carbohydrates. Therefore, meat by itself cannot completely satisfy us.

Vegetables contain some carbohydrates but not in the one-to-seven proportion. Beans come closer than any food group besides grains.

Fat is a balancing agent between proteins and carbohydrates. The body has no difficulty converting fat into either protein or carbohydrate. If the body needs energy, it breaks fat down into glucose. Glucose provides the energy. Fat is converted to protein all the time. When we work out we are converting fat into muscle protein. Conversely, protein can easily convert to fat if we eat too much protein or if we are not active.

Here's an important and little known fact. Refined carbohydrates can produce fat in the body. This means that although many foods do not themselves contain cholesterol, they can create cholesterol. Overeating can also raise cholesterol levels. Craving or eating a lot of fat is a sign that your diet is out of balance. Fat is the nutrient that is most easily converted into protein or carbohydrate in the body. If our diet approximates the one-to-seven proportion of proteins and carbohydrates, we will not crave fat. This is why it is possible to follow a macrobiotic way of eating—which is very low in fat—and feel satisfied. Grain eating is balanced eating.

Simple and Complex Nutrients—Eat One and You Will Crave the Other

There is another element to consider when attempting to balance our diet. If we eat simple minerals, such as sodium chloride (common table salt), we will naturally begin to crave complex, or denser, protein—either animal protein or very dense vegetable protein. When we eat simple minerals, meat tastes better to us. If we eat complex animal or dairy protein, we will crave simple (refined) carbohydrates. In practical terms, this means that a hamburger won't taste right on a whole-wheat bun. The complex protein of the hamburger is not attracted to the complex carbohydrate of the whole-wheat bun. Or, take the example of fish sushi. Of course, it tastes much better with white rice than with brown because, as we now understand, complex craves simple. By contrast, vegetable sushi, a simple protein, tastes better with brown rice, a complex carbohydrate.

If you eat white rice, white bread, sugar and other simple carbohydrates like potatoes, your body will begin to crave more complex protein, usually animal and dairy foods. On the other hand, if you introduce complex minerals into your diet—in the form of unrefined, white sea salt (not Celtic or gray salt, please), seaweed and pickles—you will find yourself craving more complex carbohydrates, such as whole unrefined grains, beans and vegetables. Here's a rewarding fact of macrobiotic life. Once you are eating whole grains on a daily basis, you will naturally begin to crave food that is good for you!

Refusing vegetables

As a child, I refused to eat vegetables. Lettuce and tomato (in a sandwich) were the only exceptions. My mother was an excellent cook but I didn't appreciate her skills. Food was a problem for me. Once a week I was permitted to have dinner out with my friends. These were the meals I liked best. I ate all the junk food my body could handle. Whether consciously or not, throughout my childhood I refused vegetables completely. I would eat my mother's vegetable soup only if she strained out the vegetables. I was that bad! In light of this confession, it strikes me as highly ironic that I have spent most of my adult life trying to convince other people to eat their vegetables.

Within a week of incorporating brown rice into my diet, I started to enjoy vegetables. I even began to crave them. The very food I had refused to eat for so long was suddenly appetizing and desirable. Perhaps I have even caught up with those of you who were smart enough to have eaten vegetables all along. What I'm trying to convey is the fact that the process of moving from an unhealthy diet to a healthy one occurs naturally, if we follow some simple guidelines. Once we eat brown rice and vegetables on a regular basis, our cravings for unhealthy food tend to disappear.

Seaweed seduced me next. Seaweed amazed me. I remember walking into Sanae, the only macrobiotic restaurant in Boston, on a cold day in February of 1969 and ordering hiziki on impulse. The taste was new to me, neither good nor bad, but the memory of it stayed with me. The hiziki felt right in my body and I wanted to try it again. I have grown to truly love the taste of all seaweed and the way it makes me feel. My observation is that almost everyone grows to love seaweed. For some it takes time, others enjoy it immediately. Seaweed is unique, one of the more primitive foods we have. It provides a kind of nourishment and satisfaction that few other foods offer. Perhaps it's akin to the love of raw oysters and clams that some of us develop. These are also primitive foods but seaweed is vegetable-quality and has a wider appeal. My research has shown me that seaweed was traditionally eaten by all major cultures except those in Africa, where people ate river and lake weeds instead. In our own country, some American Indian tribes traveled great distances to harvest seaweed.

Upsetting the Balance

There are various ways in which we may upset the balance inherent in the macrobiotic diet. One way is by eating too much baked or roasted or toasted food. In essence, baking, roasting or toasting is carbonizing. If you burn a piece of toast, what you are left with is carbon. Although carbon is a mineral common to all living things, the catch is that once we increase the amount of carbon in our diet through baking, toasting, roasting or burning, we automatically begin to crave more complex proteins (animal and dairy food) as well as refined grains. Excess carbon throws off the body's entire mineral balance. Cravings for strong foods, such as meat, appear; feelings of guilt and despair occur and the person to whom this is happening doesn't understand why. Too much baked, roasted or toasted food can be a recipe for disaster.

There are many tempting macrobiotic baked products available in health food stores today so it's important to keep in mind that if you eat too many of these products you will find it difficult to resist the lure of other unhealthy foods. Try to limit your intake of baked foods of all kinds, including bagels. It's okay to indulge yourself once in a while but certainly not on a regular basis.

If a little is good, a lot is not

The other most common way of upsetting the balance of the macrobiotic diet is by using too much seaweed, especially kombu. Kombu is a type of kelp that is very beneficial to health. It helps lower fat and cholesterol levels, among other things. Seaweed, including kombu, is also a good source of minerals—calcium is one of them but eating too much kombu over a long period of time can interfere with mineral absorption. To absorb minerals, we need some oil or fat in our diet and seaweed directly affects how the body utilizes oil and fat.

People tend to think that if a little of something is good for them then more must be even better, but often that's not true. Excess can lead to serious deficiency. In the case of seaweed, less is more—meaning less is better. Seaweed should be taken in small amounts but people typically increase their intake over time—often dramatically. As I just mentioned, too much seaweed can interfere with the body's ability to absorb minerals. The following is what can happen if we become mineral deficient because of an excessive intake of seaweed: in an attempt to regain its ability to absorb minerals, the body develops strong cravings for fat and protein; we begin to eat more fat and protein. Then because we feel better after eating this way, we assume it must be good for us—we must have needed more animal food. Looked at in one way, this is not an incorrect assumption. In order to overcome an imbalance, the body cries out for fat. But you can see that it would be far better not to create an imbalance at all. Be careful with the quantity of seaweed you use. It's important not to upset your body's mineral balance.

There's another problem with eating too much seaweed. One of the things the body does with fat is to convert it into sex hormones. If we decrease the body's fat content too much, in other words, if there isn't enough fat available because its absorption has been interfered with by an overuse of seaweed and salt, we invite an imbalance of sex hormones.

Highlights:

- Have at least one vegetable dish with every meal, including breakfast.

- Have a variety of vegetable dishes—well cooked, lightly cooked, pressed and raw throughout the days and weeks.

- Grains and vegetables together provide the basis of complete and balanced nutrition.

- Do not reheat leftover vegetable dishes. They lose their refreshing and nourishing qualities and leave you unsatisfied. If they have been refrigerated, take them out in advance and let them warm up naturally.

ACTIVATE AND HARMONIZE YOUR DIGESTION WITH A BOWL OF VEGETABLE SOUP AT ONE OR TWO MEALS DAILY.

Let's take a closer look at soup. Soup conditions or relaxes the digestive system and readies it to accept the meal. As I mentioned earlier, there are basically two types of soup—savory (what one ordinarily thinks of as vegetable soup) and pureed sweet vegetable soup.

Generally, savory soups, such as miso vegetable, bean vegetable or shoyu (natural soy sauce) vegetable broth, are taken at the beginning of the meal. Sweet vegetable soups are eaten throughout the meal. If you find this confusing, the safest approach is to eat your soup at the start of your meal.

All savory soups activate digestion. If a naturally fermented seasoning such as miso or shoyu is cooked into the soup, it will further aid the digestive process. Fermentation helps create good bacteria, yeast and enzymes to form a healthy environment in the intestines.

All sweet vegetable soups, being mild and sweetly creamy, help to relax, harmonize and coordinate the digestive system and its central organs—the pancreas, stomach, liver and gall bladder. When these organs are aligned, digestion is smoother. Sweet vegetable soup does not have to be pureed although it is more effective that way.

> "An old-fashioned vegetable soup, without any enhancement, is a more powerful anti-carcinogen than any known medicine."
>
> —*James Duke M.D. (U.S.D.A.)*

More savory than sweet vegetable soup

We all need a combination of sweet and savory soups, but we need about three to four times more savory soup. Serve pureed sweet vegetable soup once or twice in a seven to ten day period and eat a variety of savory soups the rest of the time. Any vegetable soup that has either miso or shoyu cooked in it is a savory soup. For instance, you can turn lentil vegetable soup into

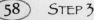

miso soup by seasoning it with miso. If you take the same soup and season it with shoyu, you create lentil-vegetable shoyu soup. Both versions qualify as savory.

Relieving Stress

Foods with a creamy texture are more relaxing and consoling and that soothing quality has a positive effect on the digestive system. During the Great Depression, sales of ice cream skyrocketed. People had no money for anything other than the bare essentials, nevertheless they bought ice cream. During really hard, stressful times, it seems we seek creamy foods for consolation. If you make sure you have the proper amount of sweet, creamy soup, you will have an easier time controlling the stress level in your everyday life. Stress hardens and tightens the digestive organs. Pureed soup helps them stay relaxed. Remember, if you're feeling nervous or pressured, it's important to take a few minutes to relax before sitting down to eat.

> "Soup puts the heart at ease, calms down the violence of hunger, eliminates the tension of the day, and awakens and refines the appetite."
> —*Auguste Escoffier*

Miso Soup

Miso soup has always been an important part of the macrobiotic diet. Recently, it's made its way into the mainstream—perhaps because it's so easy to prepare. Please consider restricting your intake of miso soup to what you make at home. The quality of miso paste used by restaurants is often very poor. Traditionally, it took at least two years to age and ferment miso properly. By artificially controlling temperature and using chemical fermentation, commercial miso can be made in one week! As an added insult, commercial miso is often flavored and dyed and may even contain monosodium glutamate (MSG), an unhealthy chemical preservative and taste enhancer. Commercial miso doesn't have any of the benefits that naturally fermented miso, available in most health food stores, has.

More is not better

It's important to have one or two bowls of soup a day. One bowl is generally enough. If you feel like having a second bowl, by all means have it. Eating soup with every meal, however, is a bad idea. As with many other food choices in the macrobiotic diet, more soup is not better. Too much soup, rather than strengthening digestion, will weaken it. As for quantity, a standard cup or small bowl sized serving is adequate. Please keep in mind that a bowl of soup by itself does not qualify as a meal—even if it contains a grain. It's important to understand that soup, whether it's miso or shoyu or sweet vegetable, does not count as a complete and nutritionally balanced meal—at breakfast or at any other time.

Which brings me to my next point. For many years, macrobiotic teaching has recommended taking miso soup at breakfast. However, it's been my observation that some people are hungry all day long if they do this and, as a result, they overeat. Why? Miso soup has a powerful capacity to stimulate digestion and when digestion is stimulated we want to eat. I now recommend taking miso soup no more than once a day at whatever meal works best for you. Experiment. Try it for lunch and, on another day, for dinner. See at which time it works best for you, at which time your leave the table feeling most satisfied.

Highlights:

- There are two main types of soup: savory vegetable soup is well seasoned and mildly salty; pureed sweet vegetable soup is mildly sweet with a pleasant creamy taste.

- Soup with a savory taste activates digestion and stimulates the appetite.

- Pureed sweet vegetable soup helps relax and harmonize the digestive system. It has a calming and consoling effect.

- Have three to four times more savory than sweet soups, i.e., one to two bowls of sweet vegetable soup in a seven to ten day period.

INCORPORATE A WIDE VARIETY OF FOODS INTO YOUR DIET.

Natural foods come in an endless variety of interesting combinations, tastes and textures. If you make an effort to try new foods and new recipes, I can assure you that your taste in food will change quickly.

Greater variety in your diet will make you feel more satisfied and will provide better nutrition as well. Start by adding a few new foods each week. The biggest mistake beginners make is to find a few foods they like and eat them over and over. Although this approach might work for awhile, in the end it leads to boredom and dissatisfaction. It is also nutritionally limited. As you become more familiar with natural foods, you will gain confidence in your ability to create satisfying, healthful and exciting meals. The more new foods you add to your diet, the more your taste for natural foods will return.

I use the word 'return' because I believe our taste for healthy food is natural. Years of eating unwisely sap our ability to enjoy natural foods. My proof is that young children love well-prepared natural foods on their first try. From time to time throughout the years, my children have been reluctant to invite their friends over for fear they wouldn't like our way of eating. Usually these friends enjoy the food so much they ask for seconds. If they don't like our food the first time, they usually come around after a few more tries.

There is far more variety available in a vegetarian way of eating than in the modern American diet. The key to success is to consciously increase variety over time. Now that so many supermarkets carry natural foods and organic produce, you can start your education there. Once you feel more confident, make a trip to your local health food store.

(Please see the Food Lists and Recipes section for suggestions.)

Styles of Cooking

Try to use a wide variety of cooking styles when you prepare your meals. The macrobiotic repertoire is extensive. For daily use, I recommend pressure-cooking, boiling, blanching, steaming, steaming with kombu seaweed (called nishime style), soup-making, stewing, quick sauteeing with water or oil, sauteeing and simmering (kinpira style), pressing and pickling. On the Occasional Use list at the back of this book, you will find baking, broiling, dry roasting, pan-frying, deep-frying, tempura (batter-dipped deep-frying) and raw food.

When planning your meals, select foods within the following categories: whole grains, soups, vegetables, beans, sea vegetables, special foods and beverages. Use different cooking methods from the above list. Keep in mind that it's best not to pressure cook vegetables. Start with those cooking styles that are familiar. If possible, take macrobiotic or natural foods cooking classes. Read cookbooks to inspire and teach you.

Vegetables can be cut in various ways. Try slicing them into rounds or half-moons. You can cut the slices straight across or on the diagonal and you can vary the thickness of the slices. Different methods have subtly different effects on the flavor and appearance of whatever dish you prepare.

Vary the kinds of seasoning and condiments you use. Use different seasonings in dishes you are familiar with and take note of how just a small change in the seasoning of a dish can produce a big difference in taste. Try seasoning that same dish with a little more or less of what you normally use. The type and amount of seasoning will each bring out different aspects of flavor and can subtly alter the consistency of a dish. Some seasonings firm up a dish, so to speak, while others have a softening effect.

It's important to vary the cooking time of vegetables. Most of us could use more lightly cooked vegetables in our diet. What do I mean by a lightly cooked vegetable? It's one that makes a crunchy sound when you bite into it. The sound should be audible to someone sitting next to you. No sound means the vegetable is overcooked. Include a combination of well-cooked and lightly cooked vegetable dishes weekly. Experiment with cooking times. Cook familiar dishes a little longer or for a little less time. And, don't forget that pickles, pressed and raw salad are part of the macrobiotic diet.

Try varying the intensity of the flame when you cook. The same dish can taste quite different depending on whether it's been cooked slowly or quickly. Many people use too much fire when cooking. It seems to be a natural tendency to turn the flame up as high as possible whether it's needed or not. Excessive use of a high flame in your cooking may make you nervous or irritable. Use a medium flame when you want to bring something to a boil. If necessary, you can always turn it up at the end of cooking. You will feel calmer and steadier as a result.

Vary the combination of dishes you use in meals. Change just one dish and you have added a new meal to your repertoire. And vary the combination of vegetables, grains, beans and seasonings you use in your dishes.

Cook your food a little longer in the winter for a warming, energizing effect. Cooking food a bit less in the summer will produce a cooling and relaxing effect.

Try to create a variety of color, taste and consistency in your meals. Variety means using many different ingredients from each of the different categories, changing the method of preparation and changing the combinations of food. Imagine what the meal will look like on the plate, imagine how it will taste. Remember that variety creates interest and satisfaction. And, never forget that food is meant to be both nourishing and delicious.

Suggestions for Planning Meals

First considerations:

- Grains and vegetables together form the basis of complete and balanced nutrition.

- All food has protein. You do not need to make a special effort to increase protein in your diet. It is nearly impossible to become protein deficient.

- A variety of vegetable foods provides the most abundant and well balanced nutrition available: minerals, including calcium, proteins, carbohydrates, fats, including omega 3, and vitamins including vitamin C.

- Beans and fish may be included in the same meal.

- Seitan, a wheat gluten product, may be cooked with grains or beans.

When planning your daily meals, try to follow the order below:

- Always decide on the grain or grain product first.

- Then choose the vegetable dish and/or dishes that complement and harmonize the grain.

- Next, decide on the soup to further complete the meal.

- Last, supplement with foods from the other categories, specifically beans, sea vegetables, seeds, nuts, fish, fruit, snacks, desserts, sweets and beverages, if you choose.

- Use these guidelines whether you are eating at home or out.

Questions to ask when planning every meal:

- What grains or grain products do I want?

- What vegetable dishes do I want?

- Will they be freshly prepared or leftover?

Questions to ask everyday:

- What soup shall I have today?

- Am I including brown rice in one of my meals today?

- Am I including a variety of well cooked, lightly cooked (meaning bright, colorful and crunchy) and raw vegetable dishes along with pressed salad?

Questions to ask when planning your weekly menu:

- What beans and/or bean products shall I have this week?

- Am I incorporating sea vegetables into my diet?

- Shall I have fish this week?

- What desserts and snacks shall I have?

- Am I getting enough variety in the other categories, including seeds, nuts, fish, fruit, mild natural sweets and beverages?

- Are my meals appealing, tasty, colorful and satisfying?

- Have I remembered to incorporate leftovers to save time on cooking?

Order of Planning Meals

	Modern Diet	Macrobiotic Diet
1. Principal foods, the centerpiece of every meal	**Protein:** Meat, poultry, eggs cheese or fish; for vegetarians: beans, soy products, textured soy protein, etc.	**Grains or Grain Products:** Brown rice, barley, millet, polenta, pasta, oatmeal, couscous, whole wheat bread, etc.
2. Main secondary foods, they complete, balance and harmonize every meal	**Starch:** Potatoes, pasta, bread, white rice or other refined grains	**Vegetables:** Well cooked, lightly cooked, pressed salad, pickles, raw salad
3. Soup with 1 or 2 meals a day	Infrequent	Miso, vegetables, lentil, pureed squash, etc.
4. Other foods throughout the week	Salads, vegetables, fruits, snacks and sweets, desserts, beverages	Beans, seeds, nuts, fish, fruits, snacks, desserts, beverages
5. Essence of a meal	Proteins, starch and beverage	Grain, vegetable and soup
6. Typical meals	Meat, potatoes and coffee Pizza and soda Pizza and beer Hamburger, fries and soda	Brown rice, steamed kale and bancha twig tea Couscous, sauteed onion and broccoli and miso soup Steamed tofu sandwich on whole wheat bread with tahini and sauerkraut, and apple juice Pasta, vegetables and tea, spring water or beer Polenta, broccoli rabe, red snapper and wine

Highlights:

- Create variety by varying the ingredients in each of the categories, changing the method of preparation and the combination of foods in the dishes you create.

- Try not to settle on a few dishes and combinations and then continually repeat them.

- Variety insures the most balanced nutrition and helps you feel more satisfied.

- All foods contain protein. The vegetable protein in grains, beans and vegetables is superior to animal protein for health.

BUY THE HIGHEST QUALITY ORGANICALLY GROWN, UNREFINED AND NATURALLY PROCESSED FOODS.

High quality organic food tastes better. It's more nourishing and strengthening to your health. Many people are willing to buy expensive cars, clothes and houses but when it comes to buying food they won't spend the extra money for the best quality. Please, don't save money on your food. Try to buy mostly organically grown food, in particular, staples like, daily-use vegetables and grains, miso, sea vegetables, shoyu, ume and brown rice vinegars and umeboshi plums etc., even if you have to travel or mail order to do it. What is not available, you can certainly supplement with commercially grown food. If most of your food is organically grown, then some unrefined and commercially produced food is not going to harm you and you will enjoy the benefits of increased variety.

That said, it's vital to remember that quality can be adjusted up or down. Here's an example of what I mean: If you think Diet (Format) is more important than Eating Habits (Content and Quality) and you want to eat organically grown, freshly hulled, pressure-cooked short grain brown rice but it's not available to you at that moment, then what do you do? Well, many people think if they can't practice perfectly, if they can't have the best food all the time, then they're not good macrobiotics. So they abandon the diet temporarily and proceed to make terrible choices. This is a pretty common response, particularly when travelling. However, if you want to eat well, you can eat well under any circumstances. If you have a health problem, the best thing to do is prepare ahead so you don't get stuck. An understanding of the controlling factors of macrobiotic practice and how to adapt to difficult circumstances is very important.

Adjusting quality

Let me explain what I mean when I say that quality can be adjusted up or down. Despite what you might think, white rice and commercially made pasta qualify as a grain and grain product. Steamed vegetables without butter are still vegetables. You

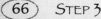

can order vegetarian vegetable soup. Will it be macrobiotic quality? No, not exactly. It may be made with potatoes or tomatoes or both but it's still vegetable soup. Remember that as long as you stick to the Format, you will be moving in the direction of health. To tell if you are becoming lax about the Format, watch for danger signals such as reading or watching TV at the table, eating or snacking while standing, not chewing thoroughly, rushing through meals, not allowing three hours between eating and sleeping and so on. If these things begin to happen and you are not alert to them, it's only a matter of time before you create an imbalance and imbalances tend to perpetuate themselves. So long as you concentrate on the Format of Meals (Eating Habits), over time your diet will become healthier and healthier. You will come to understand intuitively what you need to improve and maintain good health. But if you focus on Diet (Content and Quality of Meals), then automatically you will begin thinking in terms of good and bad, right and wrong, calcium and protein, etc., and when we think this way we get off track. It's very easy to fall into this sort of thinking. It's the way we've been taught and modern education, being so powerful, is hard to overcome.

Our goal is simply this: to have good digestion, good absorption and good circulation. After all, what is the difference between being young and being old? The answer is good digestion, good absorption and good circulation. If the food that enters the body can be digested and absorbed and the excess evacuated easily and if the blood can circulate, then we can cure ourselves of anything. We can reverse the effects of illness and unnatural aging, if we practice accurately.

Highlights:

- High quality food tastes better.

- It's more nourishing and strengthening to your health.

- Quality can be adjusted up or down.

- Buy organically grown food as much as possible. Supplement with commercially grown food when the full variety of organic food is unavailable.

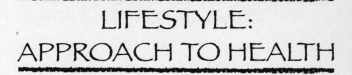

LIFESTYLE:
APPROACH TO HEALTH

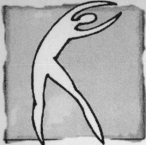

STEP 4

MAKE YOUR DAILY LIFE ACTIVE

WALK OUTSIDE FOR 30 MINUTES EVERYDAY. LIFE RELATED EXERCISE PROVIDES THE MOST BENEFIT FOR LASTING HEALTH.

I want to encourage you to make your daily life as active as you can by incorporating what I call universal exercise. Universal exercise means life-related exercise—activities directly connected to life. These are the activities that provide the most benefit and balance for all of us.

When do you think people were generally healthier—in the past when they led physically active daily lives or today when they are so exercise conscious? I always ask this question in seminars and the audience almost always responds: "In the past."

Healthy people rarely think about exercise. Their lives are so active that there's no need. They play; they enjoy and challenge themselves; they may garden, do home repairs, dance, or engage in sports. In other words, they are active but they are not formally exercising. We've been educated to think we need structured exercise. We don't. What we need is to move our bodies, to play, to enjoy ourselves physically, to challenge and stimulate ourselves. Structured exercise has a kind of hardness and rigidity about it; play has a soft and flexible quality.

Here's an analogy I like. Who is healthier—the person who eats a healthy diet or the person who eats an inadequate diet and takes supplements? My point is that since healthy people are clearly getting all the nourishment they need from their diet, the idea of taking supplements never occurs to them.

Let's apply this observation to exercise. Structured exercise is nothing more than a supplement for those people who have inadequate daily activity. In order to feel well, those who lead sedentary lives have to compensate with some kind of regular program of exercise.

Exercise versus play

Healthy children never think about exercise until they go to school where they are taught that they need to exercise. Before that they simply played and were healthy and happy. Children lose their energy only when they're told to do something they don't want to do, such as cleaning their rooms. A child's natural need to move is changing now because of poor diet. It's not natural for children to want to sit around all day and watch television. My children enjoy television but they know it's self-limiting. After awhile they are always running off to do something else. Only on rare occasions do I have to say, "That's enough TV."

The best exercise for your health is the exercise that human beings were designed to do, exercise that doesn't require machinery, gyms, or classes. Like the air we breathe, it's free of charge. I refer to walking. Walking outside at a comfortable pace with an unforced stride is the best exercise on the planet. Don't worry about cardiovascular rates and, please, don't engage in 'power walking'. The value of walking comes from the rhythmic movement—not the pace. A somewhat brisk half-hour walk every day (or two fifteen minutes ones) will keep the body fit and the spirits high. Walking increases flexibility and improves digestion, energy and cardiovascular health. It strengthens the bones and helps clear the mind and balance the nervous system. Walking is the ideal activity for everyone. It is the brown rice of physical activity, so to speak.

It's best not to think of walking as 'exercise' per se. You can think of it as a way to get from point A to point B, if you like; you can think of it as a period of time to clear your mind and let your thoughts come. The more open your mind is when you walk, the more benefit you will receive. The people who get the least out of walking are the ones who are trying to accomplish something, such as getting their heart rate up. Why? When we have an agenda, the mind closes to other possibilities. Take children as your model. Children have the best activity; they play and enjoy themselves. They don't think they're exercising or getting healthy. As long as they're playing and enjoying themselves, their minds are open.

If strenuous exercise were the panacea it is said to be, then professional athletes would be among the healthiest people in the world. Yet this is not the case. Many, perhaps even a majority, of them suffer from serious chronic injuries and other health problems. Many die young. Modern nutritional thinking says that large amounts of animal food are necessary for building stamina and keeping a competitive edge. As a result, the diet of athletes is usually high in meat, dairy products and refined carbohydrates. Athletes are given to believe that their health will not suffer since participation in strenuous sports compensates for dietary excess. Now you don't have to be a genius to understand that if you eat excessively your body will suffer the effects regardless of how much you exercise. It's a matter of common sense.

Not too long ago, I saw the results of a research study on the immune system of the professional athlete as compared to that of the average person. According to this study, the immune system of the professional athlete is weaker than that of the average person. Apparently, professional athletes are more likely to come down with colds than are those who don't compete professionally. When the body is overworked, immunity is impaired. Pushing the body beyond its natural limits in any way is not a healthy thing to do.

"The sovereign invigorator of the body is exercise,
and of all exercises walking is the best."

—*Thomas Jefferson*

Walking and balance

It's not necessary to walk briskly for a full half-hour at one time. Two fifteen-minute walks are also effective. Keep in mind that the benefits of walking come from the balancing effect of rhythmic movement on the body. We derive the greatest benefits from walking when our arms are free to swing like a pendulum. The alternating movement of arms and legs has a balancing effect on the body as a whole and on its functions as well. To be specific, this is what happens: both parts of the digestive system, the ascending and the descending colon coordinate with one another; the left lung and the right lung do the same. Both branches of the autonomic nervous system—that part of the overall nervous system that regulates breathing, digestion and, in fact, all of the body's automatic functions—are coordinated and brought into balance.

At the same time, walking helps balance the mind. When you feel anxious or worried, try taking a walk. After a short time, you will find yourself thinking more clearly and, in general, feeling better. If you are depressed, taking a walk will refresh your spirits. If you are over-tired, a walk will renew your energy. If you have too much energy, a walk will settle you down.

"Today I have grown taller from walking with trees."

—Karl Baker

Walk outdoors

Walking outdoors is far more beneficial than walking indoors. We need to be outside for one simple but compelling reason. Nature has the best circulation. Anything we do outdoors helps our circulation more than anything done inside. A walk outside in pleasant surroundings, in the woods or in a park, for example, amid grass and trees, is ideal; but even a walk on a busy city street is better than walking inside on a treadmill or track. When you walk, the quality of the air you take in is important and, as a rule, outdoor air is less polluted than indoor air. With this in mind, try to keep your home or office well ventilated. Open your windows.

Do healthy people exercise?

Let's consider an earlier statement of mine: Healthy people rarely think about exercising. The fact is that the most valuable exercise occurs as we go about living our daily lives. When we walk, shop, clean or do other things around the house, we are exercising without really thinking about it. And when we are active while doing what we enjoy—whether it's dancing, tennis, martial arts, swimming, mountain climbing or biking—we are exercising without having to force ourselves. It's important to find activities that are satisfying, challenging and stimulating. The thought should not be, "I have to do this, it's good for me," but rather, "I can't wait to get out there and do this." It's simply common sense that if you engage in activities you enjoy you will keep on doing them and never think of them as "exercise." I want to be very clear about this. I am not saying don't exercise. What I'm saying is this: Make your life active. Do whatever stimulates and challenges you. If you think it's "good" for you, don't do it.

Again, take healthy children as a model. Observe them. See how they always try to challenge and stimulate themselves. When they've had enough of something, they move on to something else.

Many people find daily exercise combined with a healthy diet to be the easiest Strengthening Health recommendation to follow. Walking is an enjoyable way to keep physically fit. If you are not already in the habit of walking, you will be surprised by the deep sense of well being that a daily walk gives.

> "All truly great thoughts are conceived by walking."
>
> —*Friedrich Nietzsche*

A Barometer

If our exercise is appropriate, our appetite for healthy food will be enhanced. Appropriate exercise helps us eat less and feel more satisfied. We can tell that our exercise is inappropriate if our craving for rich food and sweets increases, if we overeat but feel less satisfied.

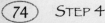

Cleaning

In more traditional times, even as recently as fifty years ago, cleaning was valued in proportion to its benefits. Cleanliness, of both person and surroundings, was said to be next in importance to Godliness. Like walking, the benefits of cleaning are universal—unless you have an attitude about it! We feel better physically and mentally when we clean. Cleaning clears the mind as it activates the body. It helps harmonize and balance our condition. Try it and you'll see.

Obesity in children

Obesity has become a major problem in the United States. Approximately forty percent of the population is overweight. "Morbidly obese" is a new term used to define that degree of obesity that is considered life threatening. There are so many obese children that even the government has been forced to take notice. Obesity in children is the cause of the current epidemic of Childhood Onset Diabetes. Obesity starts with diet. Children who are fed too many high-fat foods and sweets are less inclined to run around and play because their young bodies are too busy trying to metabolize all the excess. These children are most comfortable slumped in front of a TV set or computer for hours at a time.

Many of my children's friends are not from macrobiotic families so at our birthday parties we usually serve ice cream and other sugared foods to make their friends feel comfortable. Of course, there are always plenty of macrobiotic goodies as well. Over the past decade, I've noticed that often these children hardly touch the cake and ice cream, although my children usually eat their fair share. My explanation of this seemingly odd behavior is that these children don't find party foods to be anything special. These foods are special for my children because they don't have them very often. For their friends, however, cake and ice cream are actually everyday foods. The result is an ever-increasing rate of obesity among children.

A healthy diet creates a natural craving for activity. It's a kind of chain reaction. We need a good diet in order to be active. If we are active and if we are satisfied with our food, chances are we won't find ourselves overeating.

War and Nutrition

If we use history as a guide, we can see the effects of the decline in nutrition and activity levels by analyzing the health of the soldiers who fought in various wars. Roman soldiers were hired mercenaries. They were paid in grain, primarily an ancient type of barley, and this grain was their principal source of nutrition. Fueled by a grain-based diet, Roman soldiers conquered almost half the world. Roman generals maintained a strict daily regimen that kept their legions fit for the task of conquering strong foes, sometimes armies far larger than their own. It was not unusual for a legion to march twenty-five to thirty miles a day, each man carrying full weaponry and daily food supplies on his back. The fall of the Roman Empire followed on the heels of the widespread change in eating habits and daily activity. The Roman Legionnaires, by eating the foods of the lands they had conquered and occupied, grew lazy and gluttonous, often gorging themselves until they vomited. Banquets, at which huge amounts of food were consumed, became a feature of daily life. A downfall was inevitable.

Autopsies of young soldiers who died in action in the Korean War revealed badly clogged arteries and signs of advanced cardio-vascular disease. The medical community was shocked. The question asked was whether the government's policy of feeding soldiers a high protein, high meat diet had caused the disease. Autopsies of soldiers who died in the Vietnam War presented similar findings. In light of the evidence, it's difficult to understand why the government took so long to change its food recommendations.

Highlights:

- Walk outside to get the maximum benefit. Walking outside aligns you with the natural environment. Contact with the earth, exposure to trees and grass and to the natural circulation of air are crucial to good health.

- Walking is not exercise. It is natural movement. It creates harmony between body and mind, improves circulation and digestion and increases flexibility and bone strength.

- Walk once a day for a minimum of 30 minutes or twice a day for 15 minutes. A natural, comfortable stride is recommended.

- Imitate children and try to play rather than exercise.

- Life related activities such as cleaning, gardening, dancing, etc. provide the most benefits.

GIVE YOURSELF A DAILY BODY RUB.

Gently rub your entire body with a hot, damp, cotton wash-cloth for ten to fifteen minutes every morning and/or night. Do the rub before or after your bath or shower, but do it separately from either. The body rub is the secret of the fountain of youth. In effect, it winds back the body's biological clock. If you do a daily body rub and if you chew your food thoroughly, day by day you will become younger in body and mind.

The body rub is one of the world's best beauty treatments. People come to me for counseling with a variety of skin prob-lems—brown liver spots, white patches, blemishes and skin that is loose, dry or sagging. Often they blame these conditions on age but I believe they have unhealthy skin because they don't know how to care for themselves.

Within a few months, sometimes as little as a few weeks, these blemishes begin to disappear. Beautiful, new and younger looking skin comes shining through. Of course, your progress depends on what you eat and how well and faithfully you do the body rub. Everyone wants to look younger and healthier. Billions of dollars are spent every year on beauty creams, remedies and treatments, most of which don't work. The body rub is free and it does work.

New skin in 28 days

The skin completely renews itself every twenty-eight days. In essence, your skin is no more than a month old at any given moment. Cells in the skin are continuously dying and replacing themselves. We can renew our skin in a healthy or unhealthy way. How the skin renews itself depends on what we have been eating over the previous days, weeks and months. One of the benefits of eating well is that fresh blood is drawn continuous-ly to the surface areas of the body, stimulating the skin. If we eat healthy foods and do the body rub, we can nourish our skin on a daily basis and, as a result, our skin will become younger looking and more beautiful. Once past puberty, people of all ages can benefit from the body rub. Healthy skin is slightly shiny and moist. If your skin is healthy, your entire body perspires lightly and easily. Such skin is smooth, soft to the touch and resilient. If you push or pull it, it bounces back energetically. Healthy skin looks fresh without the aid of creams and moisturizers and is free of blemishes and pimples. The skin is an excellent barometer of overall health. I always use skin diagnosis in counseling. It tells me about the client's diet, past health problems and ability to maintain good health in the future.

Most of us take our skin for granted. We all want skin that looks young and healthy yet few of us give a thought to the skin's function. Skin is our largest organ, containing oil, sweat glands, blood vessels, nerve cells and immune cells. It has innumerable functions. It protects us from the environment, helps to keep us warm and to cool us down, produces Vitamin D, excretes toxins and, most importantly, keeps us in one piece!

The skin is our largest organ

The skin is a large, hard-working organ and one of its more significant jobs is to discharge toxins from our bodies. However, certain foods clog our skin—fatty meat, dairy products, tropical fruit, sugar, eggs, chicken, baked flour products, etc. Clogged skin means that moisture and oil cannot pass through the pores. If we eat the above-mentioned foods on a daily basis, our skin becomes dry. Most people think that dry skin is caused by a lack of oil so they turn to the common remedy for dry skin—moisturizer. Applying such a remedy will temporarily moisten the skin but then what happens? Where does the moisturizer go? It is absorbed into the fat layer of the skin, further clogging it, especially if the moisturizer is petroleum-based, like mineral oil and such saturated-fat products as coconut or palm oil.

The skin's tiny capillaries are connected to the body's large main arteries and veins through a vast network of blood vessels of ever-increasing size. It stands to reason that if these capillaries become clogged, the functioning of the circulatory system will be adversely affected. If the skin becomes so clogged that it can no longer discharge oil or moisture, then the excess fat and fluid go back into circulation through the blood vessels, looking, so to speak, for another exit. Over time, circulation will become sluggish, often to the point of putting a strain on the heart.

To help understand this process dynamically, it's useful to look at the mechanism of an event that occurs all too often in our daily lives—the traffic jam. A traffic jam on one road often clogs traffic on other nearby roads. It takes only one backed up highway exit to slow the flow of traffic and overload the entire system. Most of us have experienced, to our discomfort, what happens on a late Sunday afternoon in the summer when several exits are blocked by traffic.

Nervous System, Immune System, and Meridians

There are peripheral nerve cells in the skin that govern sensitivity and sensory perception. Since the peripheral nerve cells also send messages to the central nervous system, they influence our emotions as well. In fact, the body's entire system of nerves is affected by the condition of the skin. Imbalances in the skin affect how we respond to heat, cold, touch, pressure and vibrations. Depending on the condition of our skin, we may become over-or-under sensitive to any of the above.

The skin also contains lymphocytes, cells that are an important part of the immune system. Lymphocytes protect against viruses, bacteria and parasites. When the skin is clogged, the skin's ability to provide immunity is weakened.

Acupuncture meridians

Acupuncture meridians run under the skin and are connected to the body's internal organs. Meridians are not vessels or containers. They are energy streams, somewhat analogous to mountain streams and, as such, they have precise paths. Meridians nourish the organs and allow them to discharge excess. They help the internal organs regulate themselves and adjust to the environment. Although Western science does not acknowledge the existence of meridians, they have been known and used for thousands of years in the Far East. The ancient arts of Acupuncture and Shiatsu massage are based on and use the extensive system of meridian points.

I use meridian diagnosis extensively. It is one of my main methods for assessing someone's state of health. Meridian diagnosis gives me more information about the functioning of the body's organs and systems than any other aspect of traditional Far-Eastern diagnosis. It allows me to determine how well or poorly the body's energy is flowing along its meridians. The quality of energy flow is what tells me how the corresponding organ is functioning. The meridians actually become clogged as fatty deposits collect under the skin and as organ function weakens. When the organs are not able to adjust, they lose their ability to maintain a healthy condition. They are either losing energy or building up excess pressure.

The Pressure Valve

The skin is the body's largest organ; it is also the body's largest opening. The skin functions as a kind of pressure valve. There are many ways to release pressure. Talking, writing, physical activity, urination, bowel elimination, menstruation and sex are just some of them. Obviously, when the skin is clogged, it cannot release pressure smoothly or easily. One of the criteria of healthy skin is that its pores can open at will to release excess pressure from the body—in the same way that they open to release excess heat from the body. Our skin continually interacts with the environment in an attempt to keep the body's temperature and pressure balanced between the internal and external environments.

The body rub helps the skin function more efficiently. Clogged skin loses its ability to release internal pressure, leaving us much more adversely affected by stress. Once the skin is no longer clogged, we can release fluids and toxins the way nature intended—by perspiring freely over our entire body. It's a commonly held belief that excess energy can be released only through exercise and activity. Not true. We all know people who talk more than seems appropriate. What is not understood is that excessive talking is somewhat involuntary. It's the body's way of trying to rid itself of excess energy and stress. However, if the skin is open, internal pressure is released continuously. Once you are doing the body rub every day you will be amazed at how much calmer you are and how much better you feel.

The Kidneys, Intestines, Lungs and Liver

The kidneys are our main excretory organs. They work together with the intestines to eliminate excess from the body. The liver aids this process by detoxifying the blood. The body's normal way of discharging excess is through urination and bowel elimination. As long as the kidneys, intestines and liver are functioning efficiently, the body will not send excess to the skin. But if these organs become tired, sluggish or stagnated, the body's only choice is to send that excess to the surface, that is, to the skin or possibly to the lungs, for discharge.

One of the great benefits of the body rub is that it takes some of the strain off the kidneys, intestines, lungs and liver. By helping to clean the body, the body rub gives those organs a chance to rest and repair so they can function more easily and efficiently. It is vitally important to concentrate on the health of your skin. If the skin is unable to aid in the elimination of toxins and if the kidneys, intestines and liver are clogged and sluggish, the body has no choice but to store the excess waste which then increases the strain on your health.

Perspiration

If you don't perspire easily, this may be an indication that your skin is dry and clogged. Perspiration is natural. Many of us perspire only from certain parts of the body, like the armpits or the forehead. If your skin is functioning properly, you should perspire from your entire body. When, for instance, you take a sauna your pores should open easily. You should soon be covered in perspiration from head to toe. After the body rub becomes part of your daily routine, your skin will open and you will perspire freely, releasing those fluids and toxins that have been trapped inside.

Doing the Body Rub—Gently Rub not Scrub

I have explained the dynamics of the skin's structure and function in some detail in order to help you understand the importance of the health practice that I call the body rub. The body rub is deeply cleansing to the skin. It draws out the fat that has been collecting beneath the surface and clogging your pores.

A word of warning: If your skin looks and feels drier at first than it did before you began doing the body rub, take heart. This is good news. It's proof that you are doing the body rub accurately. Fat must gather under the surface of the skin before it can be discharged and as it gathers the skin becomes drier. I have one client who characterized the skin on her arms and legs as reptilian during the first month. Please, be patient and you will see your skin improve steadily from this point on, as she did.

The body rub is easy to do and brings immediate gratification. Some of my clients call it their morning cup of coffee—the ones who do it before bedtime report an improvement in their sleep. The body rub is easy to do. Fill your bathroom sink with the hottest tap water possible—though not scalding. The washcloth should be one hundred percent cotton, preferably unbleached or white. Fold it in half once then in half again, making four layers. Dip the cloth in the hot water and then squeeze out the excess. The cloth should be damp but not dripping. Re-dip it in the hot water as often as necessary. Rub your skin in a back and forth motion, gently and systematically. A useful image is that of the tide coming in and going out. Progress in an orderly way over your entire body. You can work from the face down to the feet or from the extremities in toward the center (just below the navel).

The areas of importance are as follows:

1. Hands, wrists, fingers (and between the fingers), feet (tops and bottoms), ankles, toes (and between the toes)

2. Face and neck

3. Armpits and groin

4. Centerline of the body, from base of neck to pubic bone; chest and abdominal areas

5. Back, including coccyx (tailbone) and sacrum

6. Elbows and knees

7. All other areas of body

If you are pressed for time, do steps 1 and 2 or 1, 2 and 3.

Do not attempt to redden your skin by using a lot of pressure. Use only the weight of your hand without pressing. Keep in mind that this is a rub and not a scrub. Your back and forth movement should be vigorous but gentle; light yet not too light. If there are parts of the skin that don't turn red, don't worry, just spend a bit more time on them. Eventually, when the overall condition of your skin improves and your circulation is responding to the treatment, your skin will redden quickly.

A word of caution: Many people have very delicate, weak skin. If your skin is thin and weak and you apply too much pressure, you can literally rub your skin off. You can think of the scabs that result as your battle scars! If you are very gentle in the beginning, your skin will become stronger more quickly. The initial process is similar to starting an exercise program. Begin slowly and build up gradually for the best results. Please be very careful when doing your face, especially the forehead and bridge of the nose. The skin along the spine is also exceptionally sensitive.

Keep Your Bath or Shower Separate

When you do the body rub, please do it separately from your bath or shower. Do it right before or right after. If you remain under the shower or in the tub water when doing the rub, you will lose too many vital minerals. Hot steam relaxes the body but since steam has the capacity to draw out minerals, too much steam can dangerous. Five to seven minutes is safe.

I recommend two methods for keeping warm if you become chilled while doing the rub, usually in winter. One is to fill the tub with hot water to just below your ankles. Then sit on the edge of the tub and proceed with the rub. The second method, the one I prefer, is to start with a very short hot shower, then turn the water off and do the rub. This allows the steam and heat from the shower to keep you warm. The bathroom will have begun to cool down by the time you are through with the rub, at which point you can finish with another very short hot shower.

Other Benefits

Another benefit of the daily body rub is that it encourages you to become more open and accepting of your body. If you really dislike doing the rub, one possibility is that you are uncomfortable with your body. In time, if you do the rub on a daily basis, your self-image will improve. You will learn to appreciate your uniqueness and you will grow to genuinely care for and respect your body. If you spend a little extra time on areas you particularly don't like, your self-image will change more quickly. Done regularly, the body rub will improve every aspect of your physical, emotional and mental health.

A word of caution: Do not use a loofa and do not use a dry brush. The purpose of the rub is to coax the pores of the skin to open in order to draw out stored fats and toxins. If you combine hot, damp heat with the softness of a wash cloth, you can easily achieve your goal. A loofa, however, even if damp, will only impede your progress. Yes, it can remove the dead outer skin, but its very coarseness causes the pores of the living skin to close tightly, sealing in fats and toxins. A dry brush may be very effective for abrading dead skin and tightening your pores, but by using one you will accomplish exactly the opposite of what you want. The body rub takes longer but it is much more effective, if your goal is to create healthy, resilient skin.

I have spent years trying to determine the best way to do the body rub and my conclusion is that strong pressure is not as effective as light pressure. As I said earlier, the body rub is a rub, not a scrub. Light pressure applied by the natural weight of the hand is what best stimulates the circulation of energy and the opening of the pores of the skin. Once the pores can open easily, they can also close easily and it is this easy opening and closing in response to both internal and external environments that is one of the hallmarks of resilient skin. If you do a daily body rub with a damp cloth and light pressure, you will discover this for yourself.

When you eat well and do the rub, in effect what you are doing is to draw a continuous supply of fresh blood to any given area. As for the face, one of the effects of improved circulation is the reduction and possible elimination of fine lines and wrinkles. Also, the rub improves muscle tone as well as skin texture so that when the facial muscles are strengthened, wrinkles tend to fade or vanish.

If you've eaten a lot of cheese and other fatty and baked foods in your life, you no doubt have deposits of cellulite in your legs, hips and buttocks. Some of my clients tell me that these parts of their bodies literally look like cottage cheese! The body rub will help break down these deposits and allow them to leave your system. Of course, if you continue to eat foods that cause cellulite, you will find yourself in an endless cycle of frustration. Now that you know the cause of cellulite, the next time you are tempted to eat cheese, just picture where it will end up. Maybe that will help you resist the temptation.

If you have very rough, red skin and feel you have to use a moisturizer, use it sparingly before going to sleep. Please don't use it in the morning. Just do the body rub. After a while, even very rough, dry skin will soften and regenerate. Except for extreme cases of very dry skin, it is unnecessary and hinders rather than helps. If used habitually, even the best quality moisturizer can clog the skin. If you must use a moisturizer, select one made with liquid vegetable oil, such as sesame or olive; avoid any oil that becomes solid at room temperature, such as coconut oil.

Highlights:

- Use a medium weight cotton washcloth. Fold it in half twice.

- Fill your sink with hot water, dip the cloth and wring it out. Re-dip the cloth frequently to keep it hot and fresh.

- Rub gently in a back and forth motion. Do not rub in circles.

- Rub gently; don't scrub. Gentle pressure yields better results.

- Do the rub separately from your bath or shower.

- The purpose of the rub is to open your pores and draw out fats and toxins. This will allow your skin to breathe naturally.

- Years of animal and dairy food, fruits, sweets, baked and fatty food clog the skin and prevent it from breathing naturally.

- The skin needs to breathe freely just as the lungs do.

Doing the body rub results in:

- An increase in the circulation of blood, lymph and energy that will improve the nutrition, oxygen flow, stimulation and health of all your organs.

- Better energy all day after a morning rub and deeper sleep after an evening rub.

- More effective release of stored toxins.

- Improved immunity to disease.

- Clearer thinking, keener memory and more optimistic outlook.

- Improved self-image.

- Increased sensual awareness.

CULTIVATE AND TAKE TIME FOR HOBBIES.

Hobbies are very, very important for good health. Yet these days how many of us have a hobby? Not many, I suspect. Hobby is a rather old fashioned word so I'm often asked what I mean when I use it. To me a hobby is something that brings an aspect of completion or fullness or balance to our lives, something we do for enjoyment—a favorite activity (not passivity)—but not what we do day to day for a living.

"To insure good health: eat lightly, breathe deeply, live moderately."

—William Londen

Let me give you an example from an older time. The Samurai of Japan were professional warriors, rigorously trained in the martial arts, who spent their lives fighting. To make sure their development wasn't overly one-sided, they also studied tea ceremony or poetry or brush painting, something very different, very highly refined, in order to make balance.

Now let me give you an example from modern life. I ask, "Do you have a hobby?" You answer, "Yes, reading." But if your job is mental, reading doesn't meet my definition of a hobby. A hobby has to be different from work, something that brings polarity and interest to your life.

I like this example: Years ago, in Science News, I came across a piece about a scientist with very interesting ideas. What struck me was the fact that a couple of times a week he and his brother got together and played guitar and sang just for the fun of it. His work was technical, highly skilled, demanding and precise. His hobby released him, balanced his work. In my view, the reason he had such interesting ideas was because he spent his free time doing something he enjoyed that was very different from his work.

> "Dare to err and dare to dream. Deep meaning often lies in childish play."
>
> —*Johann Friedrich Von Schiller*

Hobbies are a kind of self-reflection, a way of maintaining balance, a way to develop different sides of our nature. They are for our enjoyment, pleasure and satisfaction. My advice is, if you don't have a hobby, choose anything you think you might enjoy. If you find you don't like it, try something else. Often clients will tell me they don't have time for a hobby. My answer is always the same: "You don't not have time for a hobby because a hobby will enrich your life. Your practice and your health will improve if you have a hobby. Everything needs polarity. We add chopped parsley to sweet vegetable soup. The garnish brings the soup to life. In a manner of speaking, a hobby is our garnish.

Highlights:

- Hobbies make balance for the more structured and pressured areas of life.

- Hobbies help relieve stress and promote physical and mental flexibility.

- Have fun with your hobbies.

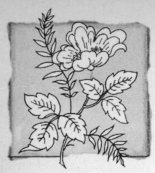

STEP 5

CREATE A MORE NATURAL ENVIRONMENT

Recharging station

What is a home? In the macrobiotic way of thinking, home is a recharging station, a place to relax, return to balance and enrich life. Therefore, we must create the healthiest environment we can so that we are nourished rather than depleted by our surroundings. The more natural the environment around us, the brighter, more refreshed and positive we feel. Then, automatically, we make better choices in all the other areas of life.

Let's say you go on a picnic. The food tastes especially delicious and you sleep more soundly that night. Why? You're out of doors in the country with congenial company, the air is fresh and usually you engage in some sort of physical activity. All this contributes to improved circulation. Whatever you do that improves your circulation creates a healthier appetite and a deeper, more restful night's sleep.

The direction modern life is taking is well beyond our control but there are steps we can take that will reverse many of its worst effects. Most of us worry about those things over which we have no control yet ignore those things we can change, things we can do every day to improve our lives. We have a choice. We can take time for our meals of grains and vegetables, stick to our daily schedule, walk, do the body rub and surround ourselves with green plants and natural materials, on our person and in our home. Each of the first five steps, if done regularly, strengthens the effect of the others. Together, the first five steps form the essence of good health. Whether we apply these principles to the life of one person, to a family, to a community or to a society, east, west, north, or south, they work. They are simple; they are unique. They worked in the past, they work today and they will work in the future. Why? Because they are based on the common sense of our ancestors but adapted to modern life.

SURROUND YOURSELF WITH GREEN PLANTS.

There was a time, not so long ago, when houseplants were considered merely decorative. Walking into a house or office filled with green plants was a pleasant, even soothing, experience, but hardly a life-enhancing one; not so any more. Plants are a necessity these days. We depend on them to clean the air we breathe, having discovered that green plants are far more efficient at removing pollutants than any machine.

Plants absorb many harmful contaminants, such as formaldehyde, benzene and carbon monoxide. Formaldehyde, one of the worst, is considered to be a contributing factor to the high cancer rate in the United States. Formaldehyde is found in many of the materials used in home building and furnishings, including plywood, particle- board, decorative paneling, floor covering, and carpet backing. It is also found in items we regularly bring into the house, such as, grocery bags, waxed bags, facial tissues, common cleaning agents, fire retardant and permanent press clothing, tobacco and cooking and heating gas.

Among the most efficient air cleaners are spider plants, golden pothos and elephant-ear philodendron. Dr. William Wolverton, formerly a senior research scientist at NASA, has calculated that fifteen to twenty of these common houseplants can clean and refresh the air in an average-sized house. Interestingly, NASA has concluded that plants become more effective at cleaning the air as pollution levels increase. It seems that in areas of low level pollution, fewer molecules come into contact with the leaf's surface so the benefits are not as great. Why are green plants so effective? They are natural generators of the negative ions in the air we breathe. Negative ionization promotes a feeling of well being, of freshness and of rejuvenation.

Negative ionization

Negative ionization increases with movement. If you walk by a waterfall, if you walk in the woods, you feel refreshed and exhilarated. The natural circulation of the water as it falls and the wind as it blows through the trees increases the amount of negative ionization in the air. When you clean a room, when you do the body rub, you are also increasing it.

An ion is a particle that can carry either a negative or a positive electrical charge. In this case, negatively charged ions are the ones we want around us. Negative ionization occurs when ions move away from the earth. It's helpful to think of negative ions as moving up and out, cleaning and refreshing everything as they go. Positive ions are those that move toward the center of the earth. Think of them as moving down and in, bringing heaviness and stagnation with them.

Any room that's not cleaned for a while will take on a dark, heavy feeling. When you open the window and pull up the shades to let in air and sunlight, when you clean the space, what you are actually doing is changing positive ions to negative ones. Fresh air, sunlight and thorough cleaning can transform any room by infusing it with refreshed energy. Being in such a room feels wonderful. Negative ionization is big news these days. Many people are buying ionizing machines for their homes. Green plants are far cheaper and far more effective. They play a significant role in promoting good health.

Large, strong plants that grow upwards are more effective than hanging plants for changing the energy in your house or office. Buy potted plants that sit on the floor. If space permits, make sure a few of them are large. A hanging plant is better than no plant at all so, if you have a space problem, resort to using one. Use as many plants as you care to, making sure there are not so many that the room looks overcrowded or movement is hampered. You don't want your guests to feel they need a machete!

Noise Pollution

One of the unsung virtues of plants is that they protect us from noise pollution. Have you ever spent time in an evergreen forest? In 1985, I was invited to teach at a macrobiotic summer camp that was held in a pine forest north of Oslo, Norway. One day, during my free time, I went for a walk in the woods. For some reason, it felt eerie being there. It took a while for me to realize that this was the first time I had ever experienced complete quiet. There was simply nothing to hear.

Plants have the ability to absorb sound. All plants can do this but evergreens are especially adept at soaking up noise. If you keep a lot of plants in the house, they will help keep the noise level down. It's easier to maintain good health in a quiet house. Doors slamming, television or music blasting and people shouting all take their toll on our health.

"One must be out-of-doors enough to experience wholesome reality, as ballast to thought and sentiment. Health requires this relaxation, this aimless life." —Henry David Thoreau

Green plants in the bedroom

The most important places in the house to keep plants are the bedroom, the kitchen and the bathroom. Many people think plants should not be kept in the bedroom. I disagree. During the day, plants give out oxygen and take in carbon dioxide. At night, they give out carbon dioxide and take in oxygen. We need more oxygen during the day, less at night, more in summer, less in winter. This natural cycle of taking in and giving out leads to greater overall oxygen intake. Having plants in the bedroom at night helps us sleep more deeply and that means we can take in more oxygen over the course of the next day. Plants in the bedroom serve to regulate the oxygen ratio so that we receive the right amount of oxygen while we sleep. As I said earlier, the body cleans and repairs itself during the night and our plants will be right there to aid in the nocturnal rejuvenation.

It's essential to have green plants in the kitchen. Ideally, the kitchen should be sealed off from the rest of the house so that cooking fumes and odors can be vented outside. Gas fumes generate a lot of pollution that spreads easily throughout the house. Green plants will help minimize their effect on our health. Water is one of the main sources of pollution in today's houses so it's best to keep green plants in the bathroom as well.

Because green plants work so diligently night and day to clean the air we breathe, they deserve proper care. Actually, houseplants require only minimal attention but they do have certain needs. They require the right amount of water at regular intervals and they must have the appropriate light. If you place a plant in direct sunlight, make certain it's meant to have a strong exposure. Different species have different needs so be sure to get some advice from the florist or consult a book. Keep your plants in clay pots so that their roots can breathe. Check every couple of seasons to see whether they require larger pots.

Highlights:

- The most important places for green plants are the bedroom, kitchen, bathroom and any other room in which you spend time.

- Green plants generate negative ionization that creates a calmer, more peaceful and refreshing environment.

- Green plants enable us to be clearer, brighter and more active during the day. Their presence promotes quiet, restful, deep sleep at night.

- Green plants are the most efficient air filtration system known, especially spider plants, golden pothos and elephant ear philodendron.

- Choose strong, upward growing plants over hanging ones.

- Choose plants that are hardy and easy to care for.

WEAR PURE COTTON CLOTHING NEXT TO YOUR SKIN.

The body runs on electrical impulses. Nutrition, digestion, immunity and our nervous system all depend on electrical impulses to do their work. Because pure cotton carries less of a static electrical charge than other material, when worn directly against the skin it helps neutralize imbalances within the body. If you have an imbalance in your nervous, immune or digestive system or in your meridians, pure cotton will help counteract that imbalance. Wearing pure cotton next to your skin is one of the quickest and easiest ways to improve and maintain your health.

Synthetics carry the strongest static electrical charge. Think of the fireworks display that occurs when you make a bed using synthetic sheets or blankets. Try making the bed with the lights off! The strong static electrical charge in synthetics interferes with the body's functioning. Synthetic fabrics make imbalances worse. Some materials that are natural to begin with go through chemical processing that produces the same effect on the body as synthetics. Rayon is a good example.

Cotton is the most neutral fabric, followed by linen, silk and wool. Silk is natural but its animal quality gives it a strong static charge. Wool is also natural but it carries a much stronger charge than cotton or even silk. It's best not to wear wool directly against the skin.

Everyone, but especially people living in modern houses or high rise apartment buildings, has an electromagnetic imbalance in his or her environment. Natural materials help lessen all imbalances. Synthetics increase, amplify and enhance imbalances. Whatever the condition of your body or your environment, it will worsen if you wear synthetics directly against your skin. If you are feeling tired, wearing a synthetic next to your skin will increase your fatigue. If you are feeling anxious, it will make you feel more anxious. Your health problems will worsen quickly if you wear synthetics against your skin.

It is especially important to wear one hundred percent cotton underwear, bras, socks and pajamas and to use pure cotton sheets, pillowcases, towels and washcloths. If you follow this simple suggestion, you will feel more refreshed and enjoy better resistance to illness. Start by replacing your underwear and socks. It's often difficult to find all cotton goods. Shop carefully and make sure to read the content labels. These days even items advertised as cotton often contain a small percentage of synthetic. When you do find what suits you, keep a record of where the item was purchased. This is helpful when it's time to reorder.

Highlights:

- Cotton is a buffer that helps neutralize imbalances in the body and environment.

- Woolens and synthetics can amplify imbalances in your body and environment.

- Underwear, socks, bras, sheets, pillowcases and towels should be 100% cotton.

- Wear cotton against the skin under clothing made from other materials.

USE NATURAL MATERIALS LIKE WOOD, COTTON AND WOOL IN YOUR HOME.

Think of your home as a recharging station. We leave home to go to work, to shop, to go to school or to play. We return to refresh, re-nourish and re-balance so we have the energy and the will to leave again. If our homes and furnishings are made from natural materials, we can recharge more effectively.

It's best to have furniture made of real wood, to chose cotton for your upholstery, drapes, curtains and wool for your carpeting. Wool carpeting is far better for your health than synthetic which, like imitation wood and plywood, is processed with formaldehyde. If you can replace the man-made materials in your home with natural ones, you will feel much more comfortable in your day-to-day life.

Natural Bedding

Try to buy 100% untreated cotton sheets. They can be expensive so keep your eye out for sales. Avoid sheets that do not require ironing. They have been treated with formaldehyde. It's far better for your health to sleep on high-quality, wrinkled but non-toxic sheets than on smooth toxic ones. It's all a matter of priorities. Reasonably priced, high-quality, pure cotton towels and washcloths are relatively easy to find. Still, it's necessary to read the content labels carefully.

A futon is the best possible choice for a mattress. Futons are generally made of cotton and their frames of wood. Make sure the futon you buy is all cotton, that it does not have a foam rubber core. If you are not ready to change your entire bed, you can buy just the futon mattress and place it over your existing mattress or box spring. Conventional mattresses are made with synthetic materials (and metal as well, in the case of inner spring mattresses) so the sooner you can replace yours with a futon the faster your health will improve.

You will enjoy the experience of having cotton close to you. In the beginning, it may take some effort to replace all your synthetic belongings but after the initial outlay of energy and money, it will be easy to replace items as they wear out. Surrounding yourself with cotton is a good health habit that will help you feel and look your best.

Transparent Building

Year ago when teaching at a seminar in Switzerland, I had the privilege of spending time in a house built of completely natural materials. The concrete was free of iron so it gave off no electromagnetic charge and the wood had been specially treated. When you were inside this house, you felt almost as if you were outdoors. It was the most transparent building environment I have ever been in. Teaching at that seminar was effortless because I was being energized all day.

Contrast that environment with that of department stores, for instance, where you are surrounded by synthetic materials and relentless fluorescent lighting. In such an environment, I very quickly become irritable. Being in man-made surroundings exhausts your body and shatters your thinking. I always feel sorry for the salespeople who have to endure this discomfort on a daily basis. Often, nowadays, there's also loud music playing. I sometimes wonder if these stores are uncomfortable on purpose. Maybe the idea is to get you to buy quickly and leave.

It's best that whatever you bring into your home be as free of chemicals and toxins as possible. Avoid using household cleaning products with high chemical content. They create their own pollution. A wide variety of excellent chemical free cleaning products are available in health-food stores, most of which are not tested on animals.

Natural food stores also have a large selection of self-care products, including cosmetics. Use these instead of conventional products that are full of chemicals detrimental to health, chemicals that are absorbed through the pores and into the body's organs where they create an additional burden on the immune system. Natural products are just as effective as—and in most cases superior to—those laced with chemicals. If you are unable to find what you need in your area, you can order from any number of catalogue companies that specialize in natural products.

Fooling the Compass

I often carry a compass with me to check out different environments. I have been amazed by some of my findings. In certain apartment buildings, my compass has been a full ninety degrees off! The concrete used in these buildings carries such a strong electromagnetic charge that when I was facing north my compass said I was facing east. Imagine how this distortion affects our health. If a compass can be thrown so severely out of balance, then we certainly can be too.

The heart of our blood is hemoglobin, an iron-containing protein. Iron is magnetic so our blood is profoundly affected by electromagnetic fields of energy. Many studies have shown that electromagnetic fields are detrimental to health. Older homes, generally built with more natural materials, tend to have weaker electromagnetic fields than new ones.

At one time, I lived in a hundred-year old Victorian farmhouse that had a very comfortable feeling. It was simply decorated with old furniture that we liked and had gotten used to. The quality of the house and the decorations helped create a feeling of comfort and well being. When friends visited, they often remarked on this. My point is that if we surround ourselves with natural materials, we can create a harmonious and balanced environment in which we can refresh and recharge ourselves.

How many times have you found yourself in physical surroundings that make you feel uneasy, even fidgety, without being able to understand why? It could be that you are sensitive enough to be adversely affected by unnatural surroundings. The excessive use of synthetics and chemically toxic materials is what creates this discomfort. Natural materials can help. Natural materials, such as wood, cotton and wool, act as a buffer, helping to lessen and balance electromagnetic interference.

Things we can control

Certain things are within our control. It's best not to use microwave ovens. Their so-called acceptable levels of radiation pollute our homes. Electric blankets are very harmful. We want to rest and recharge naturally, without interference. Electric stoves are another major source of electromagnetic radiation.

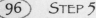

I recommend that you cook with gas. If natural gas isn't available where you live, switch from electricity to propane gas. It's easy to do and convenient to use. Cooking with electricity affects the taste and consistency of food. The flavors don't harmonize naturally and it's difficult to achieve the desired crispness. Professional chefs always choose to cook with gas.

If you have any fluorescent light bulbs in your house, replace them with incandescent or full-spectrum ones. You and your house will look much better in the glow of incandescent lighting. And your state of mind will improve. Fluorescent lighting has been proven to cause depression.

Television sets also emit harmful rays, so try to avoid spending hours sitting in front of yours. Remember that the farther away you sit from the television set, the less exposure you will receive. It's best to turn the TV off when you're not watching it as electromagnetic fields pass through walls. Lastly, please don't put a television set in your bedroom.

I am aware that the beginning of anything can be overwhelming and the practice of macrobiotics is no exception. Let's say that you have begun to eat good food in an orderly way, and have started your walking program and are doing the body rub and reaping its benefits. The next step is to surround yourself with materials that will enhance your sense of well being and contribute to your overall good health.

Highlights:

- Choose natural materials when replacing home furnishings.

- Use natural wood, cotton and wool instead of synthetic materials in your home.

- Try a futon, a natural, all-cotton mattress, for sleeping.

- Use natural cleaning products, soaps and cosmetics.

- Stop using microwave ovens and electric blankets.

- Cook with natural, propane or even butane gas. Please do not cook with electricity.

- Watch television sparingly.

STEP 6

MAKE YOUR MACROBIOTIC PRACTICE WORK

KEEPING TO THE FORMAT OF MEALS IMPROVES YOUR ABILITY TO MAKE HEALTHIER FOOD CHOICES. GOOD EATING HABITS, STEPS ONE AND TWO, ARE THE CONTROLLING FACTORS IN GOOD HEALTH.

The biggest mistake

The sixth step incorporates the essence of each of the five previous steps. The point here is that by keeping to the Format of Meals, we automatically have clear guidelines as to wise food choices under any and all circumstances, whether we're eating at home, in a restaurant, or on an airplane. As I said earlier, the biggest mistake most people make is to focus on Diet: Content and Quality rather than on Eating Habits: Format of Meals. Eating Habits are what keep us on track.

Eating home versus eating out

Food choices that are clear when we eat at home can seem murky when we eat out. When we're at home, we can choose the highest quality organically grown short grain brown rice, organic vegetables, the best quality miso and so on. If we are at the mercy of a mediocre restaurant, we might order white rice and steamed broccoli (possibly even frozen). The quality is lower, yes, but the Format is intact. We have a grain and a vegetable on our plate. Quality can always be adjusted up or down depending on where we find ourselves. Of course, the degree of the adjustment depends on our condition. We must ask: "What can my health afford at this time? How liberal can I be?"

As simple as this might sound, most people see little or no connection between meals at home and meals outside the home. At home they take care to make good choices but when they eat out they often throw away the guidelines, meaning the Format of Meals and choose whatever appeals to them. This is a serious mistake. The Format is what helps us maintain our direction toward health. If, however, we believe Content and Quality are more important than Format and we can't get organic short grain rice, the temptation is to abandon the Format as well. Once we create a separation in our minds between what we eat at home and what we eat outside, it follows that we begin to see food in terms of black and white. We think, "I ate something I shouldn't have, I'm off the diet, I'm in trouble, I can never eat out, this is too hard." But, really, if we focus on the Format wherever we are, we will automatically make the wisest choices possible and we will continue to move in the direction of health.

The second biggest mistake

Let's look at maintaining the direction toward health from another angle; structure (another word for Format) versus variety. The second biggest mistake most people make is to allow the structure, which should be tight, to become loose. Once that happens, the need for variety diminishes and eventually changes to a pattern of repetition, a pattern that directs us away from health. If the legs of a table are loose, the table can be said to have a wobbly structure. It can barely support itself. If we remove the legs altogether, the table will collapse completely. Or to use Nature's model once again, the sun rises and sets everyday, a phenomenon that is part of the structure of the universe. If the sun doesn't rise or set, it's all over for the planet. In the same way, once we let the structure or Format go we set ourselves on a path away from health.

Here are the main danger signals:

- You don't sit down and take time for your meals.

- You do other things while eating.

- Your mealtimes become irregular.

- You stop having a grain and vegetable with every meal.

How does this work? Let's say you want to have lunch at twelve-thirty, no later than one o'clock, but you're too busy to eat. By the time you do eat, your appetite is completely altered because your blood sugar has fallen. Low blood sugar means that in order to feel satisfied either you have to eat more than usual—in other words, overeat—or you have to have something sweet. It follows that, once having eaten a late lunch, you have no appetite for dinner at the regular time. If you keep to your regular dinnertime but eat less than usual, an hour or two later you'll want a snack. Or, instead of dinner at six, let's say you decide to eat at eight-thirty. Either way, you won't have three full hours between dinner and bedtime since you have to go to bed at a reasonable hour in order to get up early the next morning. You don't sleep very well that night (no one sleeps well on a full stomach). It's difficult to get up the next morning and, when you do drag yourself out of bed, you don't feel refreshed. You can see how one change in the structure or Format inevitably leads to another and how, in the end, these changes will lead you away from health.

Although having a grain and vegetable with every meal comes under the heading of Diet, there is an overlap with Format. The meal you sit down to eat must qualify as a meal, meaning it must contain a grain or grain product and a vegetable. When you stop having both a grain and a vegetable with every meal, most commonly that meal is breakfast and it's the vegetable that disappears from the plate. If you've reached this stage, you can pretty much assume you've begun to lose your direction. You're getting way off track.

Balance and imbalance perpetuate themselves

One of the guiding principles of life is that balance perpetuates itself. And, as you might suspect, imbalance perpetuates itself as well. As you let go of more and more of the structure, you start to feel more and more pressure. You might believe the build up of pressure comes from having to market, prepare and cook the food or from the pressure of having to eat at a regular time—but I don't think so. I think the reverse is true. The usual pattern is that you feel rushed so you begin to rush your meals. The more we rush our meals, the more rushed we feel. Sitting down and taking time for meals actually eases pressure. If you think of a meal as a time for recharging, reorienting and regaining balance, if no matter how stressed you feel you take the time to sit down, eat slowly and chew well, when you finish eating you will feel refreshed and calm. Any decisions you make in this frame of mind are bound to be wiser than those made under pressure.

Some people find it helpful to think of chewing as a form of meditation, somewhat like breathing practices. The result in both cases is heightened mental and emotional clarity and a feeling of deep calm. Remember, it's important to come to the table prepared to chew. Before you sit down, ask yourself. "What are my priorities?" If good health is one of them, then take time for your meal, eat your food slowly and chew it well.

Structure Versus Variety

Let's go back to structure versus variety. I said earlier that when the structure becomes loose, the need for variety diminishes—or we could say, tightens—and eventually repetition replaces variety altogether. In effect, polarity is reversed. What do I mean by this? Let me start with a basic premise: the more we seek variety, the more nutrition we get from our food. If we eat the same few foods over and over again, eventually not much happens. If someone repeats the same thing over and over again, eventually you stop hearing what is being said. It goes in one ear and out the other. It's no different with food. In one end and out the other—without much benefit.

Unfortunately, often we don't notice that this is happening. It's difficult to be aware of what we're eating day-to-day. Food is the closest thing to us so we don't have the advantage of perspective. We think we have variety—we eat blanched, steamed and sauteed vegetables daily; we eat different grains, oatmeal, brown rice, millet, barley—where's the repetition in all this? Every morning we have oatmeal and steamed kale; for lunch we have rice and blanched broccoli and cabbage; for dinner, miso soup, rice with sesame seeds, sauteed mixed vegetables, pressed salad with nappa cabbage. Isn't that variety? No. It's repetition. Taking several dishes and repeating them day after day after day is repetition. Having blanched broccoli and cabbage every day for lunch is repetition. Having oatmeal for breakfast every morning is repetition.

Appetite is stimulated by variety. Variety also creates satisfaction. If we lack variety in both ingredients and preparation, we don't feel satisfied with our food and so we overeat at mealtimes and snack before bed.

Highlights:

- Good eating habits, steps one and two, are the controlling factors in good health.

- Good eating habits increase your ability to make healthy choices.

- When traveling or eating out, keep to the format of grains and vegetables as the basis of a meal. Quality can be adjusted up or down. White rice or commercial pasta is a better choice than going without a grain.

- Commercial vegetable soup is a better choice than no soup at all.

KEEP A DAILY MENU BOOK TO HELP YOU BECOME MORE OBJECTIVE ABOUT YOUR MACROBIOTIC PRACTICE.

Underlying everything in this book so far is the basic question, how do we keep moving in the direction of health? Keeping a menu book—or a journal, if you prefer to call it that—is the best way I know of. It's very difficult to be aware of what we're doing day to day, especially with regard to diet. As I've said before, food is the closest thing to us so it's hard to be objective. The power of a menu book is that it lets you see if you are really getting enough variety.

Enter the date, time and menu for every meal, snack or nibble that passes your lips along with a brief comment on how you felt that day. Review your menu book every so often and reflect on its contents. It's difficult to be objective when you are entering information. Objectivity comes later. In this way, you will know whether or not you are getting variety. Keeping a daily menu book takes the guesswork out of tracking the changes in your health. (It's not necessary to include recipes, although you may if you wish.)

Your menu book can be as simple or as detailed as you care to make it. Some people keep track of their daily functions as well as their daily food—bowel movements, bed time, sleep patterns, moods, and so on. Looking back, you can see how you were feeling physically, mentally and emotionally on any given day. Then you can begin to correlate what you ate or did on a particular day with how you felt that day. For instance: I did this and I felt really good—my thinking was clear, I ate this and I didn't feel very well, I did this and I was irritable, I did that and I was really tired. You can't learn this sort of thing in school. How certain foods, patterns and behaviors affect you can only be self-taught. If you write just a sentence or two every day, that should be enough to jog your memory and help you discover whether you are really doing what you think you're doing. I can't stress enough the importance of keeping a menu book. It's one way to measure how serious your commitment is to improving and strengthening your health.

I must confess I've never really kept a menu book but in the past, during the years when I was teaching several times a week, I kept a kind of journal. I entered the outline of every lecture I gave along with some comments, no matter how often I lectured on the same topic. It's interesting to look back over these journals. There are times when I thought my condition was good and my thinking orderly but my journal shows otherwise. Or, looking back at other periods when my notes indicate that my condition was off, I can see by the outline of my lecture that my thinking was very clear and orderly. The point is that when you're in the throes of doing something, it's nearly impossible to be objective. But when you look back you can often see the truth.

One final comment on this point: You might think you don't need to do this, you're an experienced cook, you don't need to improve your cooking. Let me assure you that even experienced, long time macrobiotic cooks keep menu books. I can guarantee that if you keep one your practice will improve, as will your cooking. Objectivity is the key. You can see where you've fallen short or gone overboard.

Highlights:

- Keep a hard or spiral bound book in your kitchen to record your menus and snacks.

- Keep notes on your activities, symptoms and general feelings.

- Refer back to previous days, weeks and months to see any patterns that emerge from your practice.

- Keeping a daily menu book is one of the best ways to improve your practice and discover your mistakes.

- Such a journal allows you to evaluate your practice and its benefits more objectively.

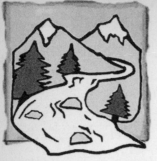

STEP 7

CULTIVATE THE SPIRIT OF HEALTH

The seventh step is the one that completes the other six, the one without which the other six remain mechanical and, in a sense, external to us, animated by willpower rather than love. What is too often missing from current macrobiotic practice is the spirit of health itself. It's taken me a long time to work out how to convey the essence of this spirit—one that is inseparable from the theory and practice of macrobiotics. Lacking this spirit, we can never make the transition to lasting health.

Please bear with me as I repeat once again: Health is a direction, a condition we move toward day by day throughout life. Sickness is also a direction. Depending on the totality of our eating habits, diet and daily lifestyle practices, we move in one direction or the other. It should be no surprise then that if we follow the macrobiotic guidelines accurately, we move toward health. If we ignore them, we move toward sickness. Let me state something unequivocally: Health is a condition we grow into throughout our lives. This is a very important point. Today, the most commonly held belief is that we start out in life with a certain amount of health—call it our capital—that we spend as we age until, in a manner of speaking, we are bankrupt. Now, to believe that aging is a fate that brings, among other things, the loss of bones, teeth, beautiful skin, flexibility, memory and the ability to enjoy and fully participate in life—that this fate is as sure as death and taxes—is a very heavy burden to bear. Yet this belief is so strong that everyone who can afford to carries the financial burden of a lifetime of health insurance.

Is this kind of deterioration really the human fate? I don't think so. Is the aging process I have just described based on a natural model of aging—of living in harmony with nature—or is it simply the experience of those who live an anti-natural lifestyle? I think you know the answer. Let me assure you that it is not natural to deteriorate with age. If you look at nature's model—take for instance, trees—what do you see? Once the aptly named 'mighty oak' has grown to fullness, then seedlings sprout and when these seedlings need more light and more space to continue growing, the oak passes on. In other words, when the oak has fulfilled its destiny, it moves on.

> "A wise man should consider that health is the greatest of human blessings, and learn how by his own thought to derive benefit from his illness."
>
> *—Hippocrates*

In the past, people readily moved on when they had had enough of life. It was that simple. (In fact, the novels of the nineteenth century are filled with death-bed scenes involving characters who, having reached this point, put their affairs in order, paid their debts, said their farewells to family and friends and either sat down or lay down and died.) They chose the time and place of their death. They died not of sickness but because they had had enough of life. Some of you might have had parents or grandparents who were able to do this. Odd though it might seem to us, it's really no different from anything else we've had enough of in life. No matter how much we enjoy something, eventually we reach a point of satiation where more isn't going to add to the experience. In fact, it may well detract from it. We can have the best conversation, the best meal, the best vacation, whatever. Still, sooner or later, we get to the point of fullness and satisfaction. We've had enough. It's time to move on. It's a sign of spiritual maturity to know when that time is.

For the first eighteen to twenty years after birth, we grow our bodies. At that point, the body should stop growing—in terms of weight as well as height. Our natural weight is achieved somewhere between the ages of sixteen and twenty. People new to macrobiotics are sometimes quite heavy. The prospect of losing weight appeals to them but often they lose more than they are comfortable with. I always ask, "How much did you weigh when you were sixteen? How much did you weigh when you got your first driver's license? That's your natural weight and that's probably what you'll end up weighing." They become alarmed. "That's too thin," they say. No, it's not too thin. Let me explain. As I said, we spend the first part of life growing the body. At birth, the body is not completely formed. The nervous system is not fully developed nor are the lungs, immune system or bones. We take the next sixteen to twenty years to grow these after which we stop growing physically and begin to grow mentally and spiritually. That is, we begin to grow our consciousness.

"Dwell not upon thy weariness, thy strength shall be according to the measure of thy desire."
—*Arabian Proverb*

Health itself has three aspects: physical, mental and spiritual. Physical health is the foundation of mental and spiritual health. When we have good vitality, good energy, then we sleep well. If we sleep well then we are alert and our memory is excellent. We don't anger easily. We are filled with a deep sense of joy and appreciation. On the other hand, with limited physical vitality, sleep isn't usually sound or refreshing, memory is unreliable and there is a tendency to become easily irritated. Worst of all, joy and alertness are lost along with feelings of gratitude for life itself.

As I said, the first part of life is devoted to the growth of the body and the creation of a high degree of physical health. Physical health is the foundation for the growth and nourishment of mental and spiritual health. When you look at traditional societies, you see that they valued their elders for their life's experience and their ability to guide younger people. Think about it, if the elders were incapable of guiding their own lives because of impaired memory and physical debilitation, how could they guide anyone else? Why would anyone seek them out? The answer is that the memory of the elders didn't deteriorate. On the contrary, it increased with age. Their patience with life itself, their joy, their appreciation for all of life, their understanding of the relationship between difficulty and happiness—all these increased and flowered as they aged. Just as the flower represents the culmination of the growth process of a plant, the final maturation before passing on to the next stage, so old age should be the flowering of our life on earth.

What we refer to when we talk about health these days— health being merely an absence of serious illness—is a very recent model. The world's health began to deteriorate at the time of the Industrial Revolution but the definitive turning point was World War II.

It's most important that we reexamine our definition of health itself. We must ask ourselves what health is and what we need to do to develop it so that old age is once again a flowering. One thing that does change with age is that we become less interested in sensory experience and more interested in social matters. We become more interested in discovering for ourselves the meaning of life—that is, in discovering what we came here to do so that we can complete the task, so that one day we can honestly say we are satisfied, we have had enough of this life.

> "And man dies and is buried, and all his words and actions are forgotten, but the food he has eaten lives after him in the sound or rotten bones of his children."
>
> —*George Orwell*

I'd have to say, based on my years of counseling so many seriously ill older people, that most of them never did what they really wanted to with their lives. They were waiting until retirement to make their dreams a reality but once retired they found they didn't want to do anything. Almost inevitably what followed was a very rapid physical and mental deterioration. It's almost axiomatic that doing what we really want to do day to day is what nourishes life and health. Those activities that we never grow tired of, that we don't want to retire from, that, in effect, never end for us, are life and health giving. Work we love is a form of play. If we live this way, then, like the elders of traditional eras, when we are ready to hand the baton off to someone else, we will do it with gratitude and in the spirit of adventure.

Let's start here: We are all guided by our consciousness. If our consciousness keeps telling us that we are going to get sick and die, then that's generally what happens. But if our consciousness is constantly guiding us toward health, health is what we get. A genuinely healthy person has more energy, more vitality and a greater interest in life as he or she ages. I have seen it over and over. We all have this capacity.

I have spent the greater part of my adult life trying to create the guidelines that will help those who are interested achieve the kind of health I have been describing. Let's examine the seventh step or last guideline in more detail.

BE OPEN AND CURIOUS AND CULTIVATE AN ENDLESS APPRECIATION FOR ALL OF LIFE.

Everyone likes to look at healthy children. Why do you suppose that is? For one thing, their faces are open and clear, not closed and clouded with conceptual thinking, bad experiences and heavy responsibilities. Since they don't have to get up in the morning and work at jobs they hate, their faces reflect an incredible openness and sense of curiosity. This openness is the source of their energy. When you look at a child, you see bright freshness, the same sort of freshness you see when you look at a healthy plant. A healthy plant is one that is getting the proper nourishment. The soil, water, sunlight, breeze, temperature—everything is suitable. We can say the plant has good nourishment and good circulation. When we look at a healthy child, we see the same thing. Healthy children can eat very, very little or they can eat a lot or they can eat very simple food and still grow very well. The reason for this is that they have good digestion, meaning they are able to absorb nutrition very efficiently from whatever amount of food they eat. At the same time, they have excellent circulation. They can go out in the coldest weather with almost no clothing on and they don't feel the cold. Their circulation is so good that they have no hardness in their bodies. You can bend children, twist them like pretzels and the more you do this the funnier they think it is.

> "Gratitude is the heart's memory."
>
> —*French Proverb*

We can see this very clearly by looking at plants. If their nourishment, temperature or circulation is off, plants react very quickly by losing their freshness. If you over water they become limp and lifeless, if you under water they become hard, dry and inflexible. What I am trying to convey with this analogy is that openness or freshness, curiosity and appreciation mean that we are connected to nature, connected to life itself—or to God, if you prefer to say it that way. The benefits of a good connection are good nourishment and good circulation.

Experts today are concerned about children's lack of activity. As I mentioned earlier, we are in the midst of a nationwide epidemic of juvenile obesity as well as juvenile diabetes. Parents are being urged to take their children outside and play with them. Isn't this a strange idea? When I was a kid, our parents couldn't get us to come indoors even for meals. It was a constant battle. There is something really wrong when kids don't want to play. Before children were told that they had to exercise to be healthy, they had the best exercise in the world—play—but once they were introduced to it as a concept they no longer wanted to exercise at all. Today, children's minds are infected with unhealthy ideas from many sources. Their minds are full of junk ideas, their bodies full of junk food. The inevitable result is a loss of openness and circulation. All of a sudden it's too cold or too hot to go outside. Minds and bodies close and become inflexible and our children no longer have the openness, freshness and curiosity they had just two or three years earlier.

The way for anyone to recover openness and curiosity is to consciously practice gratitude and appreciation. This practice opens the mind and the heart. When we complain, blame and criticize, we close our minds. You can say we close ourselves off to life itself or to nature or to God. Let me give you an example of what I mean. In the early years of my practice, I had a client with colon cancer who had refused surgery. This man, who was a concentration camp survivor, had an iron will. For a year and a half, he ate everything I recommended. After the first nine months, he went to have a check up with the doctor who had diagnosed him. When the doctor couldn't find any trace of the cancer, he assumed he had misdiagnosed the case. My client continued to practice macrobiotics for another nine months. Then one day I got a phone call from his son. He told me his father had begun to eat other sorts of food and was having health problems again. I suggested that his father return to my original recommendations. The son called back and told me his father was refusing to eat the macrobiotic way, that he would rather die than continue to eat the food. And that's what happened. He ate the macrobiotic way for eighteen months but during all that time he failed to develop a sense of gratitude or appreciation for what had been given to him. I know it sounds harsh but I have seen this kind of response again and again in my thirty odd years of counseling. The man with colon cancer was so strong willed that he would have eaten sawdust for a year and a half, if I had recommended it. Yet because he didn't develop a deep sense of appreciation, the food that gave him back his life never became delicious to him.

"To speak gratitude is courteous and pleasant, to enact gratitude is generous and noble, but to live gratitude is to touch heaven."

—*Johannes A. Gaertner*

Let's say there's a man you like, someone you appreciate, and that person does something you're not too crazy about. You don't drop him. Since you're fond of him and appreciate his qualities, you don't give too much weight to what he's done. You cut him some slack. However, if you aren't open to him to start with and, as a consequence, can't appreciate his finer qualities, then what he's just done becomes a huge impediment and chances are you'll drop him altogether.

What I'm getting at is this: Appreciation shows openness. If we're open to someone, we see more and more of their good qualities. If we're closed, we see more and more of their negative ones. Appreciation is an expression of our openness to life, our willingness to receive life itself. And that openness manifests itself day to day in a deep interest in and curiosity about life, about everything—food, friendship, love, sex, adventures, travel, history and so on.

> "Take only memories, leave nothing but footprints."
> —Chief Seattle

BE FLEXIBLE AND ADAPTABLE IN YOUR PRACTICE.

There are only two ways I know of that will help you keep your practice flexible and adaptable. One is to establish a deep connection with the source of life and renewal that is the natural world. You can do this by practicing the seven steps really well. The other is to keep in touch with new developments in macrobiotic thinking. Everything changes over time. Everything adapts or dies. Nothing is fixed in cement, including macrobiotics. In today's rapidly changing world, adaptability and flexibility are more important than ever before. Those people who have been practicing for five, ten, twenty years and haven't adapted their ways of cooking and eating to the changing conditions of life inevitably get into trouble. We have to look carefully at what we're doing on a daily basis. If we can't recognize an imbalance in ourselves—and it's very hard to see in oneself—then we should seek guidance.

Of course, the degree of flexibility you can permit yourself depends on your health and the circumstances in which you find yourself. Health is freedom. The better your health, the more relaxed you can afford to be socially. If your health can't afford it then no matter what the situation or circumstance is, it's better not to mess around. If you're healthy, one binge won't harm you but if you have a serious health problem and you've been practicing well, one binge can cause devastation. If health were money and you were making five hundred dollars a week, then a thousand-dollar car repair would represent serious damage to your financial health. But if you were making ten thousand a week, it would be no big deal.

Ideally, of course, it would be wonderful if everyone could eat very carefully day to day and be adaptable and flexible socially when appropriate. To be able to do this depends on your degree of health. My hope is that you make yourself healthy as quickly as possible so you can do what you want. Let me repeat that health is freedom. People think that freedom produces more freedom but I don't agree. I prefer to use words like order or structure rather than discipline but the meaning is the same. Freedom rests on and comes out of discipline.

> *"When you're finished changing, you're finished."*
> *—Benjamin Franklin*

Where is it most important to exercise discipline, in our Eating Habits or in our Diet? Do we exercise discipline by making sure we sit down to eat, take time for meals, have a grain and vegetable with every meal, etc. or do we exercise it by thinking, I can eat this, I can't eat that? The answer, of course, is we apply discipline with respect to our Eating Habits. For most people, diet is not discipline. If we enjoy the food, we look forward to eating it. In my book, that's not discipline.

One last point: Please try to be flexible and adaptable not only in your own practice but also in your dealings with your children, partners, relatives and friends.

DEVELOP A STRONG WILL AND THE DETERMINATION TO CREATE YOUR OWN HEALTH.

The will to create enduring health has to come from within. No matter how loving, generous and helpful family and friends are this is a gift they cannot give us. My long-time observation is that people who want to become well do just that. I am always being asked, "Can macrobiotics help cure my illness?" But the question should be, "Can macrobiotics help me cure myself?" It's the person who determines the outcome, not the disease, just as it's the person who determines what illness he or she will get. Have you ever wondered why is it that we get one sort of illness and not another? Based on my counseling experience, I can tell you that we get only that type of illness or disease that perfectly fits our nature. Why should this be the case? Think about it. Becoming ill is an indication—an alarm-bell, in some cases—that we've gotten way off-track, that we are seriously out of balance. And we each get out of balance in our own particular way. The type of illness we contract tells us what we need to learn about ourselves in order to get back on track.

> "Valor consists in the power of self-recovery."
> —Ralph Waldo Emerson

If we are open and appreciative, then we can understand the significance of the illness in our lives and we can change. If not, then we will just go on repeating the behavior that brought us the illness in the first place. Those who have overcome a terminal illness all say the same thing. "My illness was the best thing that ever happened to me. It changed my life."

> "It is idle to say that men are not responsible for their misfortunes."
> —Samuel Butler

Some years ago, I invited a young couple from Philadelphia to be part of a panel discussion I led after a lecture I gave at a natural foods convention. The husband had had testicular cancer many years before and had refused to have his testicle removed surgically. In the beginning, he didn't practice macrobiotics consistently well. He'd visit me, practice well for a while and then he'd ease up. Well, the cancer spread, it put pressure on his kidneys and he nearly died. He had to have serious, heavy-duty chemotherapy. He recovered but his doctors claimed that the spread was due to my interference in his medical treatment. He said, "No, he gave me good advice but I didn't take it. This was entirely my fault." At any rate, his doctors told him he would be sterile. It's important to know that throughout this long ordeal he never gave up practicing his version of macrobiotics. I assured him that if he could bring himself to practice really well, he could overcome the sterility. I'm happy to tell you the couple has three strong, healthy children. During the panel discussion, his wife said, "My husband's cancer was the best thing that ever happened to us. Without it, we wouldn't have found the macrobiotic way of life and we wouldn't have had such wonderful children," one of whom is a highly gifted pianist. I was used to hearing such remarks from the person who'd been ill but this was the first time I had ever heard—and from a spouse—that macrobiotics was the best thing that had ever happened to an entire family.

"Who is strong? He that can conquer his bad habits."

—Benjamin Franklin

BE ACCURATE IN YOUR PRACTICE.

Accuracy is a spiritual practice, plain and simple. If we are accurate in our practice, it means that we have the ability to devote ourselves to something, to be with something completely without any separation, without any distraction. It means that we understand the value of small things and how the small relates to the large, how the part relates to the whole. So often it's the little things in life that make a difference. It's been said, and rightly so, that God is in the details. For example, we can make the most wonderful dish in the world but if we don't season it properly, it won't come to life, it won't taste delicious even though everything up to the point of seasoning was done well. The point at which we add salt to a dish determines the degree of flavor the dish will have, whether it will taste salty or sweet. In this case, accurate timing is crucial.

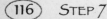

To practice the macrobiotic way of life accurately means you must pay attention. You must give your undivided attention to sitting down to eat, to chewing well, to getting variety, to doing the body rub and so on. To pay attention means to be there mind, body and spirit—with no separation—in the moment you are doing these things. Accuracy is something that is learned by example and training very early in life. If we haven't had the good fortune to learn it then, we have to work hard to recover our ability to be accurate. And this ability is often the deciding factor in whether or not we recover. Accuracy is a condition of body, mind and spirit. It is a spiritual practice, not a mechanical one.

"The near explains the far. The drop is a small ocean."
—*Henry David Thoreau*

My father was a diamond setter. He taught only two people, my cousin and myself, although there were many others who wanted to learn the trade at that time. When you apprenticed yourself to him, your first job was to sweep the floors, sweep them well and sweep them endlessly because the bits of precious metals and gems that had fallen to the floor in the course of the work had to be recovered. Almost everybody failed the sweeping test. They couldn't or didn't want to learn to sweep accurately. If they couldn't be accurate when sweeping, my father wouldn't teach them anything more. He'd say, "They're not worth teaching. They can't even sweep the floor." His thinking was, if you're going to do something, do it well or don't do it at all.

Accuracy regarding the seemingly smallest and most meaningless tasks, that is, the willingness, the patience and the ability to do the most meaningless thing fully and completely is a quality that fewer and fewer people seem to value. Yet those living in spiritual communities, such as monasteries, willingly undertake the most menial chores and do them with appreciation and joy, understanding that it is through this work that they will grow spiritually. If you find it difficult to be accurate, then perhaps one way to develop this quality would be to take on more and more menial tasks and do them with a full heart. Try it and see. The more accurate and precise you can be in your practice the more you will receive from your efforts—across the board.

Now although I use the word accurate, often the client will substitute the word strict. I want to be clear about this—accuracy and strictness are two entirely different qualities. For one person, to eat simply is accurate. For another, to eat widely is accurate. For some, to eat in restaurants is accurate. For others, to stay away from restaurants is accurate. Accuracy and strictness are not connected in any way but often when people hear accuracy, they interpret it as strictness. Strictness is a straight path to rigidity and rigidity is a condition of hardness.

> "Good timber does not grow with ease.
> The stronger the wind, the stronger the trees."
>
> —*J. Willard Marriott*

Please, think about the meaning of the word accuracy and about how to be accurate. Accuracy implies flexibility and adaptability according to the circumstances. It's impossible to be accurate if you don't know what the requirements are. Part of learning to be accurate is to find out what the requirements are. They might involve attending classes, reading books and so on—in other words, taking the time to find out whatever it is you really need to do to develop that quality of mind, body and spirit we call accuracy.

CREATE A GOOD SUPPORT NETWORK.

The need to create a good support network is greater than ever. So much of what we have to learn can only be transmitted personally. In the old days, serious students had the attractive option of living in study houses. Most of us who are still actively teaching macrobiotics spent time living in study houses—six months, a year, five years—where we lived and breathed the subject. We roomed together, studied together, played together, cooked for each other and ate together. The focus of life in the study house was to deepen one's understanding of all aspects of the macrobiotic way. The sort of education we got was very different from what most people have access to today.

Short of a study house, what can you do to create a support network? All of us need to find ways to be around healthy macrobiotic people. If among your friends or acquaintances there's a macrobiotic family that knows how to practice well, try to spend time with them. If you live in a major city, chances are you can find a macrobiotic community there. Information of this sort is sometimes posted on health food store bulletin boards. If you live in a more remote area, the best thing you can do is to attend major macrobiotic programs at least a few times a year—even if you have to travel great distances to get to them. Doing this will make all the difference in your practice and your health. Being in a group of people who are healthy really picks you up. There's a group dynamic that works to everyone's benefit. Your health will improve more rapidly than it would on your own no matter how well you are practicing. And if your practice has deteriorated because of isolation, you will be inspired to clean up your act.

When I first established my school, The Strengthening Health Institute, the program consisted of two non-residential weekends. I soon realized that for the program to become more effective, it had to be residential. Students need to feel they are part of the school; they need to be involved at every level. I wanted to recreate the experience I had had of living and breathing macrobiotics and that's very difficult to achieve if students arrive in the morning and leave in the evening. Macrobiotic study programs generally offer a traditional learning structure. As with martial arts schools, there is usually a mix of new and experienced students, something along the lines of a one-room schoolhouse where different grades are taught together and a bit like the structure in large families where the older children typically help the younger ones.

Please do whatever it takes to create your network. Without one, it is much harder to move in the direction of health.

LEARN TO COOK WELL.

Finally, learn to cook well. I can't emphasize this enough. Macrobiotic food has a bad reputation. Many people think the food is terrible. Well, it all depends on your experience. If your first macrobiotic meal is bad, it's easy to dismiss all macrobiotic food. It's useful to remember that the world is full of bad cooks—no matter what sort of food they are preparing. And macrobiotics is no exception. However, a bad macrobiotic meal may be worse for you than an ordinary meal! Unrefined, organic grains and vegetables carry more ki (energy) than their counterparts. They store more energy and vitality. If macrobiotic food is well prepared, it nourishes you more than ordinary food. The down side is that if it's poorly prepared, the effects stay with you longer. We can say that macrobiotic cuisine has the potential to be the most delicious or the most dreadful of any cuisine.

"Good cooking does not depend on whether the dish is large or small, expensive or economical. If one has the art, then a piece of celery or salted cabbage can be made into a marvelous delicacy; whereas if one has not the art, not all the greatest delicacies and rarities of land, sea or sky are of any avail."

—*Yuan Mei*

Please remember that no one's cooking is perfect. Perfection is not the point and it's not our goal. Even the best cooks falter. What we strive for is the ability to express ourselves accurately through our cooking, in the same way that artists express themselves accurately through their art. I don't think anyone will dispute that cooking is an art. What's more, cooking is a form of art that creates life. And what is art if not the expression of one's personal vision of life on earth. Our ability to stay with macrobiotics—and not just to stay with it but to embrace it with a full heart, to choose it enthusiastically over all other ways of life—depends a lot on how well we learn to cook. Whether we cook everyday or periodically, we should know how to cook well.

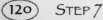

The more we know about what it takes to put a delicious macrobiotic meal on the table, the more appreciative we can be of the efforts of others.

I've observed over the years that there seem to be two different takes on the subject of macrobiotic food. The basic one, and the one I subscribe to, is that the food itself is delicious. Our job is to learn how to bring out its natural taste, color and texture, using simple ingredients and traditional techniques. Simple ingredients and proper techniques are all we need to produce a delicious, satisfying meal. In this style of cooking, modeled after Japanese temple cooking, seasoning, spices and oil are used sparingly but to great effect.

Then there's the other approach. The thinking behind it goes something like this: "I'll put up with this food for now but once I get healthy I'll be able to eat the good stuff. I'll be able to eat more widely." There's nothing wrong, per se, with eating widely or with eating simply. It all depends on our condition. What's wrong is the implication that once we can use more oil, once we can cook with herbs and spices, once we can eat tropical fruits and vegetables, then we'll be practicing the 'real' macrobiotics and our food will be truly delicious.

This is simply not true. Furthermore, what's particularly unsettling about this approach is the belief that the simple meals we eat day to day are not the most delicious, satisfying, nourishing or fulfilling ones we can have. I think this is a dangerous approach. There is nothing more delicious than well prepared brown rice or miso soup or blanched steamed or sauteed vegetables. On what do I base my assertion? The test for me is how many days in a row, how many years in a row I can eat a particular food and continue to find it delicious, satisfying and nourishing. Now we've all gone to fine restaurants and thought the food was incredible and said, "That was one of the best meals I've ever had." I translate such a statement to mean that if we eat such a meal once a year, it does taste that delicious. But if we eat it once a month, it tastes a bit less delicious. And, if we eat it weekly, well—you get the picture. If we eat such a meal everyday, it's a safe bet that we won't be able to stand the sight or smell of it after a while. It's just too much. It's an assault on our senses. What this means to me is that such a meal is not truly delicious. Of course, from time to time, it's wonderful to have such a meal. It's a bit like describing someone as a great person and then saying you can only take that person in limited doses—which is quite different from saying, "This is a great person, someone I really want to spend lots of time with."

"Cook it with pleasure - eat it with joy."
—*Clarissa Dickson Wright*

The problem is that learning to bring out the truly delicious natural taste of food without relying on such things as herbs and spices to take up the slack takes more time, patience, sensitivity and skill than other sorts of cooking. Here's a generalization I think is valid: Since I've been involved in macrobiotics, I've observed that you can divide people practicing macrobiotics into two groups. Those who, when they come up against a problem, look inward and those who, in the same circumstances, look outward. The ones who look outward don't last. (Actually, they don't last at anything.) Let's say they become dissatisfied with one or more aspects of the macrobiotic way of life—the philosophy, the healthcare, the spirituality, the cooking, whatever—it doesn't really matter. Eventually we all meet with resistance. We come up against the brick wall of ourselves, so to speak. It's part of living. And then we have two basic choices. We can look outward and think, "Someone out there has got to get me past this, someone has got to help me or I'm out of here." Or we can look inward and think, "I already have the means to help myself. If I just stick with this, I'll get through it." Inevitably, we all arrive at that point of resistance in our cooking. We find ourselves thinking, "Is this all there is, no more ingredients, no more choices?" I can guarantee this will happen to you. When it does, if you stop and ask yourself, " What can I do to make my food more delicious and exciting?" a new dimension will open up and you will be able to take your cooking to the next level. This is how the process of growth works.

If we look outside ourselves for the answer, then we relinquish the ability and the power to create or change our lives.

This doesn't mean that we have to do everything by ourselves, that we can't ask for help. At one time or another, we all need guides but we are the ones who choose them. We are the ones who decide when we need help and for how long a time. We might decide we need shiatsu massage or that we want to improve our cooking or that we have to learn more about macrobiotic philosophy so that we can better help ourselves. This frame of mind is the polar opposite of someone who thinks, "This person is going to help me" or "that person is going to save my life." That's dependence. We are moving toward freedom.

Everything I've been saying comes down to this: A healthy person is self-reliant and self-sufficient. My approach to life has always been that if we're here we already have what we need to take care of all our problems. We might require help from time to time to get past a rough spot or to have something pointed out to us or to give us a little push. But, still, it's up to us to choose what we want to do and how much energy we want to give it. It's up to us to take the initiative in our own lives. In other words, it's up to us to behave in a self-sufficient manner and that means not waiting around for someone or something 'out there' to come to our aid. Modern life encourages dependence. Part of the macrobiotic journey or adventure—for it is an adventure—is to free ourselves of that dependence by learning to develop our own healing ability and, through struggle, to gain the power to create the life we want.

"A good cook is like a sorceress who dispenses happiness."

—Elsa Schiaparelli

For many of us today, the principle issue is one of health. The challenge is how to create good health so that we are free to live our lives. But let's not forget that health is guided by spirit. And it is in the spirit of macrobiotics to look at the challenges and difficulties that come our way as gifts. For it is in meeting challenges and in overcoming difficulties that we begin to develop the power to heal ourselves, the power to build the life we want. To be truly healthy, we have to embrace the spirit of health.

Which brings me to my final point. Although the spirit of health has many components, it would be a grave mistake to forget the totality. We cannot separate one part from any of the others without destroying the whole. For instance, leaning to cook well requires accuracy but it also it requires flexibility and openness. You see what I mean. Macrobiotic thinking differs from modern thinking in both its ability and its willingness to look first at the whole and only then at the parts out of which that whole is formed. If we look at life through the lens of macrobiotics, it becomes clear that each part of life is dependent on all the other parts. It follows then that if we destroy any part of life, we contribute to the destruction of all of life. On the brighter side—or what used to be called 'the side of the angels'—if we enhance any part of life, we help to refresh all of life.

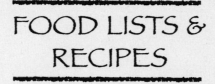

FOOD LISTS & RECIPES

SUGGESTIONS FOR GETTING STARTED

Look for:

- Organically grown foods where possible.
- Whole grains instead of refined grains and brown rice instead of white rice.
- Whole-wheat flour, bread, and spaghetti. When buying whole-wheat bread, make sure that it is made from 100% whole-wheat flour. (Some commercial brands are just glorified white bread.)
- Fresh vegetables for every meal.
- Unrefined white, sea salt.
- Unrefined oils, such as sesame, corn, olive, sunflower, or safflower oils.
- Jams without sugar.
- Fruit juices without sugar.
- Rice syrup and barley-malt syrup as natural sweeteners instead of sugar.
- White-meat fish over meat and chicken.
- Proteins such as beans, tofu, seitan, and tempeh instead of meat and cheese.
- Non-stimulating teas and grain coffees.
- Sea vegetables for your cooking. These vegetables are sources of valuable nutrients, including calcium, beta-carotene, and vitamin B-12 that help reduce cholesterol, rid the body of toxins and strengthen immunity.
- Foods from the FOODS FOR REGULAR USE list.

FOODS FOR REGULAR USE

Whole Cereal Grains and Flour Products
Use a variety with every meal

Whole grains

Use often

Short-grain
brown rice

Medium-grain
brown rice

Barley

Millet

Wheat berries

Corn-on-the-cob

Whole oats

Rye

Buckwheat

Long-grain brown
rice (hot climates)

Sweet brown rice

Cracked and flaked grains

Use occasionally

Pounded sweet rice
(mochi)

Barley grits

Bulgur

Cracked wheat

Couscous

Rolled oats

Steel-cut oats
(Irish oats)

Corn grits

Cornmeal (polenta)

Rye flakes, barley
flakes, or other flakes

Other traditional
grains (amaranth,
quinoa, etc.)

Flour products

Use occasionally

Whole wheat
noodles

Japanese wheat
noodles (udon)

Japanese thin wheat
noodles (somen)

Japanese buckwheat
noodles (soba)

Bread (unyeasted
sourdough whole
wheat or whole
rye or whole corn)

Puffed wheat gluten
(fu)

Boiled wheat gluten
(seitan)

Pancakes
(homemade)

Vegetables
Use a variety with every meal

Use often

Green leafy:
Bok choy
Carrot tops
Chinese cabbage
Collard greens
Daikon greens
Dandelion greens
Kale
Leeks
Mustard greens
Parsley
Scallions
Turnip greens
Watercress
Round:
Acorn squash
Broccoli
Brussels sprouts
Buttercup squash
Butternut squash
Cabbage
Cauliflower
Hokkaido pumpkin
Onion
Pumpkin

Use often

Rutabaga
Turnips
Shiitake mushroom
Root:
Burdock
Carrots
Daikon
Dandelion roots
Jinenjo
Lotus root
Parsnips
Radish
Sweet vegetables:
Carrots
Cabbage
Daikon
Onion
Parsnip
Pumpkin
Winter squash
Broccoli
Cauliflower
Leeks

Use occasionally

Broccoli rabe
Celery
Chives
Cucumber
Endive
Escarole
Green beans
Green peas
Iceberg lettuce
Jerusalem artichoke
Kohlrabi
Mushrooms
Pattypan squash
Red Cabbage
Romaine lettuce
Salsify
Snap beans
Snow peas
Sprouts
Summer squash
Wax beans

Beans
Use no more than once a day

Use often

Azuki beans
Black soybeans
Chickpeas (garbanzos)
Green or brown lentils

Use occasionally

Black-eyed peas
Black turtle beans
Great Northern beans
Kidney beans
Lima beans
Mung beans

Use occasionally

Navy beans
Pinto beans
Soybeans
Split peas
Whole dried peas

SPECIAL FOODS

I've classified the following foods in this category because they have been used for hundreds of years in various cultures and have unique taste, nutritional, and health qualities.

The special foods can be used as a regular part of your diet.

Soybean products

Use occasionally

Dried tofu
Fresh tofu
Natto
Tempeh

Seasonings for cooking

Use often

Barley miso (mugi), aged 24 months

Brown rice miso (genmai)

Shoyu (naturally fermented soy sauce)

Unrefined white sea salt

Seasonings for cooking

Use occasionally

Brown rice vinegar
Ginger
Garlic
Mirin (sweet taste)
Tamari
Umeboshi plum
Umeboshi paste
Umeboshi vinegar
Wasabi (horseradish)
White miso

Sea vegetables
Use often

Toasted Nori Sheet
Wakame
Kombu

Sea vegetables
Use occasionally

Agar-Agar (kanten)
Dulse

Beverages
Drink a comfortable amount for thirst

Bancha twig tea (kukicha)
Bancha leaf tea (green tea)
Roasted barley tea

Roasted rice tea
Spring water
Filtered water

FOODS FOR OCCASIONAL USE

Fish
2 to 3 times a week

Choose from non-fatty white-meat fish
or salmon occasionally

Carp	Halibut	Trout
Cod	Red snapper	Salmon
Flounder	Scrod	
Haddock	Sole	

Seeds And Nuts
1 to 2 cups a week each

Seeds and nuts may be used in cooking, as garnishes with a variety of dishes, and as snacks. Seeds and nuts may be eaten dry or oil-roasted. Pumpkin seeds, and occasionally sunflower seeds and walnuts, may be eaten raw.

Seeds	**Nuts**
Pumpkin seeds	Chestnuts
Sesame seeds	Almonds
Sunflower seeds	Peanuts
Roasted tahini or sesame butter	Walnuts
	Pecans
	Nut butters

Sweets and Sweeteners
Use as snacks or in cooking

Barley malt	Diluted apple juice or cider
Brown rice syrup	Diluted grape juice
Rice and barley malt candies from health-food stores	Pure maple syrup (use sparingly)

Fruits
Cooked, dried or fresh, seasonal Northern climate fruits
2 to 3 times a week

Ground fruit
Blueberries
Blackberries
Cantaloupe
Honeydew
Raspberries
Strawberries
Watermelon

Tree fruit
Apples
Apricots
Cherries
Grapes
Peaches
Pears
Plums
Raisins
Tangerines

Other Foods and Seasonings

Mild herbs and spices
Natural sauerkraut
Cucumber-brine pickles
Horseradish
Lemon

Toasted sesame oil
Light sesame oil
Olive oil
Corn oil
Safflower oil

Beverages

Amasake
(sweet rice beverage)

Diluted apple juice,
grape juice, and
other fruit juices
(not tropical)

Beer (microbrewed)

Carrot juice (and other
vegetable juices)

Herbal teas

Sake

Soy milk

Sparkling
mineral waters

Wine

USE SPARINGLY OR AVOID

Baked flour products and refined grains
Muffins
Crackers
Cookies
Pancakes (commercial)
Rice cakes
Chips
Baked pastries
Puffed whole
 cereal grains
Popcorn
White rice
Commercial pasta
Commercial whole
 wheat or rye bread

Vegetables
Artichoke
Asparagus
Avocado
Bamboo shoots
Beets
Eggplant
Fennel
Ferns
Ginseng
Green or red pepper
New Zealand spinach
Okra
Potato
Rhubarb
Spinach
Sweet potato
Swiss chard
Tomato (fresh
 or sun-dried)
Taro potato (albi)
Yams
Zucchini

All tropical nuts, including:
Brazil nuts
Cashews
Hazelnuts
Macadamia nuts
Pistachio nuts

All tropical fruit, including:
Banana
Coconut
Dates
Figs
Mango
Papaya
Pineapple
Citrus fruit

AVOID AS MUCH AS POSSIBLE

Red Meat
Beef
Lamb
Pork
Poultry
Chicken
Duck
Turkey
Dairy Foods
Milk
Butter
Cheese
Yogurt
Ice cream

Sweeteners
Artificial sweeteners
Brown sugar, molasses
Carob
Chocolate
Fructose
Fruit sweeteners
Honey
Sugar substitutes
White sugar

Beverages
Artificial beverages
Carbonated waters
Cold drinks, iced drinks
Coffee (regular or decaf)
Distilled water
Hard liquor
Regular tea
Stimulant beverages
Tap water
Other
Lard
Margarine
Artificially processed foods

STYLES OF COOKING

Use often

Pressure cooking
Boiling
Blanching
Steaming
Steaming with kombu (nishime-style)
Soup-making
Stewing
Quick water sautéing
Quick oil sautéing
Sautéing and simmering (kimpira-style)
Pressing
Pickling

Use ocassionally

Baking
Broiling
Dry-roasting
Pan-frying
Deep-frying
Tempura (batter-dipped
 deep-frying)
Raw food

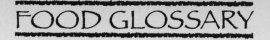

FOOD GLOSSARY

Our goal was to keep these recipes simple. Wherever possible we have used familiar ingredients. We understand that any change in diet requires a rethinking of old food habits; having to learn about new food products presents an additional challenge. You will find, however, that many of the recipes do include unfamiliar ingredients, products that have such strong health benefits and are so delicious that it is important to become familiar with them and use them on a regular basis. The following is a list of those items:

Miso: Miso is a remarkable food. Once you get into the habit of using it, you will wonder how you ever managed to cook without it. Miso is a paste made of fermented soybeans, grains, water and sea salt. Miso is a source of essential amino acids, vitamin B 12 and minerals. Miso soup acts as an antidote to stress by relaxing the nervous system. There are many different types of miso from which to choose. The best kind for daily use is barley miso, also called mugi miso. The other is brown rice miso. Sweet white miso is lighter in taste and will add variety to your meals. Many more types of miso are available and it is fine to use other varieties occasionally; however, for optimum health use barley or brown rice miso on a regular basis. It is important to use only miso that is natural (traditionally made) and that has been aged for at least two years. Make sure to buy this product at a reputable health food store.

Shoyu: Everyone has used soy sauce, either at home or at a Chinese restaurant. Shoyu is simply traditionally made, naturally fermented soy sauce. What distinguishes it from regular soy sauce is the fact that it is not chemically processed. It is made from soybeans, wheat, sea salt and water. Use shoyu with a light touch. Do not drown your food in it! Shoyu should be used only for cooking, not at the table. Keep it in the kitchen. Overuse leads to intense thirst and a strong craving for sweets. A small amount of shoyu goes a long way.

Umeboshi vinegar: This vinegar is extracted from the Japanese ume plum. Sorry, I know we promised to keep it simple but this vinegar is so delicious and so taste- enhancing that we thought you should become familiar with it. The use of umeboshi vinegar will help lighten your digestion.

Udon noodles: These are Japanese wheat noodles. They have a nice light flavor and are free of chemical preservatives.

Sea Vegetables: kombu and wakame: Sea vegetables are the plants of the sea. They are packed with vitamins, minerals and trace elements.

We hope that you find this chapter helpful and that you enjoy using these recipes. Once you become familiar with the ingredients, you will find it easy to improvise and come up with variations of your own.

Good health is built on the choices we make daily. Don't forget, every day, at every meal, make sure to have both a grain and a separate vegetable dish. Take one or two small bowls of vegetable soup daily. You will be amazed at how much better you will feel.

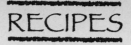

RECIPES

The recipes in this book were contributed, and in some cases created, by Susan L. Waxman.

PRESSURE COOKED BROWN RICE

Ingredients:

Short or medium grain brown rice, rinsed

Sea salt or kombu, rinsed

Water

Ratio: 1 cup of rice to 1 1/4 - 1 1/2 cups of water

Soaking:

Place the rice in a bowl and add the water.

Cover with a bamboo sushi mat and let the rice soak for 6 – 8 hours or overnight.

Preparation:

• Place the soaked rice along with its soaking water in a pressure cooker.

• Add either a pinch of sea salt or a postage stamp-sized piece of kombu seaweed.

• Lock the lid into place on the pressure cooker. Light the burner and adjust the flame to medium. Place the cooker on the burner and bring it to full pressure. Then put a flame deflector under the cooker, lower the flame and cook for 50 minutes.

• Remove from the flame and allow the pressure to come down naturally.

• Remove rice from the cooker with a wooden paddle.

• Place rice in a serving bowl and cover with a sushi mat or towel.

 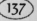

MILLET & SWEET VEGETABLES

Ingredients:

1 cup of millet, washed

1 - 1 1/2 cups of sweet vegetables, diced
Choose from a variety of sweet tasting vegetables, such as: leek, cabbage, onion and winter squash, etc.

Ratio: 1 cup of millet to 3 - 3 1/2 cups of water.

Preparation:

- Dry roast millet in a skillet until it gives off a nutty fragrance.
- Layer the sweet vegetables in the bottom of a heavy pot.
- Place the roasted millet on top of the vegetables.
- Add the water and a pinch of sea salt.
- Cover and bring to a boil over a medium flame.
- Place a flame deflector under the pot, lower the flame and simmer for 40 minutes.
- Gently mix the vegetables and grain together, being careful not to mash.
- Place in a serving bowl and cover with a sushi mat.

FRIED RICE WITH LEFTOVER RICE

Ingredients:

1/2 of a small onion, diced   Light sesame oil

1 stalk celery or a carrot, diced   Sea salt

2 cups of leftover rice   Shoyu

Preparation:

- Lightly heat a pan for 10 - 20 seconds and add 1/2 - 1 teaspoon of light sesame oil.
- Tilt the pan so the oil disperses evenly. Be careful not to let the oil burn. If it begins to smoke, discard it and start over.

- Add the diced onions and begin to sauté. When onions are fully coated with oil, add a tiny pinch of sea salt and sauté for about another 3 minutes

- Add the celery and sauté another minute.

- Add the diced carrot and sauté for one minute more.

- Add a small amount of water to the pan. This helps prevent the rice from sticking.

- Add rice and mix with the vegetables.

- Cover and let simmer for 1 - 2 minutes.

- Season very lightly with shoyu, blend, cover and simmer for 4 - 5 minutes.

- Remove from pan, place in a serving bowl and cover with a sushi mat.

Optional:

Mix in toasted nori or nori flakes.

Add a little pepper or grated ginger juice.

NOODLES & BROTH

Noodle Ingredients:

1 packet of udon (wheat) noodles or soba (buckwheat) noodles

Noodle preparation:

- Fill a pot with water and bring to a boil.

- Add the noodles and cook until tender. To test for tenderness, break a noodle in half. When the color and consistency are the same throughout, the noodles are ready.

- Empty the pot into a colander and run cold water over the noodles, then put the noodles back in the pot, cover them with cold water and empty again. Repeat this process 3 times or until the noodles are cool. Japanese noodles can be salty. Rinsing them removes excess salt.

Note: You may use the "shocking" method to cook the noodles. Bring water to a boil, and add the noodles. Pour cold water into the pot to stop the boiling, then allow the water to come back to a boil. Repeat this process several times or until the noodles are ready.

Noodle Broth

Broth ingredients:

2 inch strip of kombu, rinsed

1 or 2 dried shiitake mushrooms

1/8 teaspoon of sea salt

1/3 of a medium-sized onion, sliced in half moons

1/3 cup of thinly sliced leeks or nappa cabbage

4 1/2 - 5 cups of water

Broth preparation:

- Place the water in a large pot.
- Add the kombu and the shiitake mushrooms.
- Bring to a boil. Boil for 2 minutes then remove the kombu.
- Add the sea salt and cook 2 - 3 minutes.
- Add the onions and simmer 5 - 7 minutes.
- Add leeks or nappa.
- Season with shoyu and let cook another 5 minutes.
- Place the noodles in a bowl and cover them with broth.
- Garnish and serve piping hot.

Optional:

Add a small amount of mirin at the end of the cooking.

Add fresh tofu cubes after seasoning with shoyu.

Garnish suggestions (use only one or a combination):

thinly sliced scallions, toasted nori, toasted seeds, grated ginger, grated daikon

COUSCOUS WITH FRIED SEITAN AND VEGETABLES

Ingredients:

1 cup of couscous

1/3 cup of carrot, diced

1/3 cup of celery, diced

1/2 cup of onion, diced

1/2 cup of diced seitan (wheat gluten)

3 cups of water

Sea salt

Shoyu

Sesame or olive oil

Preparation:

- Place the water and a pinch of sea salt in a pot and bring to a boil.
- Put the couscous in an earthenware or pyrex bowl.
- Pour the boiling water over the couscous to just cover.
- Cover the couscous with a plate and let sit for 5 minutes.
- Heat a skillet and add the oil.
- Add the onion and sauté.
- Add a pinch of salt.
- Add the celery and seitan and continue sautéing.
- Add the carrots and sauté a bit longer.
- Add a small amount of water.
- Season the vegetables with a few drops of shoyu.
- Fluff up the couscous and mix with the vegetables.
- Season with a few more drops of shoyu and gently blend.
- Place in a serving bowl and cover.

Optional:

This dish may be seasoned with a little ume vinegar instead of additional shoyu.

Chopped parsley or nori flakes may be added.

Substitute cooked chick peas for the seitan.

POLENTA

Ingredients:

1 cup of yellow cornmeal

Sea salt

3 1/2 - 4 cups water

Preparation:

- Place the water and a pinch of sea salt in a pot, cover and bring to a boil over a medium-high flame.

- When the water is boiling, remove the lid and slowly add the cornmeal.

- Stir until all the water has been absorbed into the polenta. Stirring is important to prevent clumping.

- As the polenta thickens, it will begin to bubble.

- Continue stirring until the polenta clings to a spoon.

- Cover the pot and simmer for 30 - 40 minutes.

- Place a flame deflector under the pot.

- Serve the polenta soft, or place in a Pyrex dish to cool and set.

- Once set, the polenta may be cut into squares, deep-fried, pan-fried or grilled.

Note: This dish is delicious served with beans or sautéed vegetables.

SOFT RICE USING LEFTOVER BROWN RICE

Ingredients:

Leftover brown rice

Water

Ratio: 1 part rice to 2 - 3 parts water

Preparation:

- Place the leftover rice in a pot and add the water.
- Cover and bring to a boil on a medium-low flame.
- Place a flame deflector under the pot, lower the flame and simmer until the rice has a slightly creamy, porridge-like consistency.
- Add more water if needed.

STEEL CUT OATS

Ingredients:

Steel cut oats

Sea salt

Water

Ratio: 1/4 - 1/3 cup of oats to 1 cup of water

Preparation:

- Place the oats in the water, add a pinch of sea salt and bring to a boil.
- Lower the flame, cover and place a flame deflector under the pot.
- Simmer on low for 40 minutes.

- Stir half-way through cooking time.

Note: For rolled oats follow the above recipe but cook only about 7 minutes or until soft and creamy.

MILLET & SWEET VEGETABLES

See the earlier Millet & Sweet Vegetables recipe, but use the ratio of 1 cup of millet to 4 - 4 1/2 cups of water.

SOUP

BASIC MISO SOUP

Ingredients:

¾ - 1 inch piece of wakame sea vegetable per serving

2 - 3 pieces of thinly sliced root and/or round vegetables per serving, such as: onion, cabbage or carrot.

Leafy greens, finely sliced

1/2 - 1 level teaspoon of aged barley miso per cup of water

Scallions, finely chopped

Preparation:

- Soak the wakame until soft. Discard the soaking water and chop the wakame into small pieces.

- Place the chopped wakame in a pot, add the water and bring to a boil over medium-high flame.

- If using onion, add it first and boil without the lid to cook

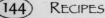

off the strong flavor. This will sweeten the onion.

- Add the root and round vegetables.
- Cook the vegetables for 4 -5 minutes, until they become tender.
- Add the leafy greens.
- Remove a little broth to a small bowl and dissolve the miso in it.
- Add the miso to the boiling broth.
- Gently stir the soup and then reduce the flame to low.
- Simmer for 4 minutes on a low flame
- Garnish each serving with chopped scallions.

SIMPLE LENTIL SOUP

Ingredients:

1 inch-square piece of kombu sea vegetable

Diced onions, celery, and carrots

Lentils, sorted and washed

Chopped parsley or scallions

Sea salt

Shoyu

Note: 1 cup of lentils yields 4 - 5 servings

Preparation:

- Place the kombu in the pot, then layer in the celery, onion, carrots and lentils.
- Add water to cover the lentils by 1 - 2 inches.
- Cover the pot and bring to a boil on a medium flame.
- Reduce the flame to low and simmer for 45 - 50 minutes.
- Add more water as the lentils expand.
- Continue to cook, covered, until the lentils are soft.
- Add a pinch of sea salt and cook for 7 - 10 minutes.

- Season the soup with a little shoyu and cook for 5 - 7 minutes more.

- Garnish with chopped parsley or scallions.

Options:

For a thinner soup, use slightly less lentils or increase the amount of water.

For a richer taste, deep fry a slice of bread, cut it into croutons and garnish.

PUREED SWEET VEGETABLE SOUP

Ingredients:

Use a combination of sweet-tasting root, round, and leafy vegetables. Include onion often because of its sweetness and ability to combine well with other vegetables.

Sea salt

Shoyu

Preparation:

- Wash and dice the vegetables.

- Place the diced onion in a pot with 2 - 3 inches of water and bring to a boil.

- Add a tiny pinch of sea salt and simmer for 5 minutes.

- Layer in the other vegetables.

- Add 1/4 – 1/2 teaspoon of sea salt, cover, and bring to a boil.

- Reduce the flame and simmer for 20 - 25 minutes until the vegetables are tender.

- Puree, preferably using a hand mill.

- Return the pureed soup to the pot. Add more water, if necessary, to achieve the desired consistency.

- Season with a few drops of shoyu and simmer 5 minutes on a medium-low flame.

- Garnish each serving with chopped parsley or scallions.

Note: This soup is meant to be sweet. Adding salt at the beginning of cooking brings out the natural sweetness of the vegetables. A little shoyu used at the end creates a deeper, more relaxing effect.

VEGETABLE DISHES

NISHIME or WATERLESS COOKING

Ingredients:

1 square-inch piece of kombu seaweed, soaked

A variety of root and round vegetables, cut into large, thick chunks

Sea salt

Shoyu

Note: This dish works best with a heavy pot and lid.

Preparation:

- Place kombu and soaking water in a pot.
- Layer the vegetables in the pot from yin to yang or light to heavy.
- Add enough water to cover the bottom of the pot, about 1/4 inch.
- Sprinkle a tiny pinch of sea salt over the vegetables, cover and bring to a boil over a medium flame.
- You will hear the water boiling and you may see some steam escape from the pot. (Try not to lift the lid).
- Lower the flame and simmer for 20 to 30 minutes, or until the vegetables are tender.

- Remove the lid and lightly season with a few drops of shoyu.

- Replace the lid, pick up the pot and shake it gently, using a circular motion, to blend in the the shoyu.

- Return the pot to the stove and cook for another 4 - 5 minutes.

- Remove the pot from the flame and let it sit for a few minutes, with the lid on, before placing the vegetables in a serving dish.

QUICK SAUTEED VEGETABLES

Ingredients:

Medium-sized onion, sliced in thin half moons

Root and/or round vegetables, thinly sliced or cut into matchsticks

Leafy green vegetables, thinly sliced

Light sesame oil

Sea salt

Shoyu

Note: This dish cooks quickly. Sautéed vegetables should be bright, colorful and crunchy.

Preparation:

- Gently heat a skillet for a few seconds and then add the the oil.

- Heat the oil over a medium-high flame. The oil should be hot, but not smoking

- Tilt the pan so the oil spreads out evenly and just coats the bottom.

- Sauté the onions until they are coated with oil. Please use wooden cooking utensils.

- Add a tiny pinch of sea salt.

- Add a small amount of water, followed by the root and/or round vegetables.

- Sauté for 1 minute.

- Add the leafy greens and mix in.

- When the colors begin to deepen, season the vegetables with a few drops of shoyu and blend. Remove the vegetables from the skillet and place in a serving dish.

BLANCHED VEGETABLE SALAD

This light and colorful dish is a combination of root, round, and leafy green vegetables. They are meant to be bright in color and crunchy in texture.

Ingredients:

Vegetables from at least 2 of the 3 following types:

Leafy greens, thinly sliced

Round vegetables, quartered and sliced thinly

Root vegetables, cut into matchsticks or thinly sliced

Sea Salt

Water

Note: An oil skimmer (a fine mesh hand held strainer) is useful for removing vegetables from the water.

Preparation:

- Half-fill a pot about with water. Add a tiny pinch of sea salt.

- Bring the water to a boil over a medium flame.

- In an open pot, blanch one vegetable at a time, starting with the mildest in taste and lightest in color. When you add the vegetables to the boiling water, the boiling should stop.

- When the color brightens, remove the vegetable from the pot and place it on a plate. Cover with a sushi mat and drain off any excess water.

- After the water returns to a boil, add the next vegetable.
- Repeat the above for each vegetable.
- Allow the vegetables to cool and gently mix them together in a bowl.
- Cover with a sushi mat until ready to serve.

QUICK STEAMED GREENS

Quick steamed greens are a lightly cooked vegetable dish. Steamed greens should be bright, crunchy and a little deeper in color than blanched greens. Use only one type of leafy green per serving. (Broccoli may be considered a leafy green.)

Ingredients:

A leafy green from the "regular use" list, leaves and stems separated and thinly sliced.

Note: You will need a bamboo or stainless steel steamer basket.

Preparation:

- Place 3⁄4 - 1 inch of water in the bottom of a pot and insert a steamer basket.
- Cover the pot and place it over a medium flame.
- When the pot is filled with steam, add the stems to the basket, cover and steam for 20 - 30 seconds.
- Add the leaves, cover and continue steaming.
- Steam for 1 - 2 minutes, depending on the texture of the vegetable.
- Remove the greens from the basket and place in a serving dish. Cover with a sushi mat.
- If desired, sprinkle 2 - 3 drops of shoyu on the greens and toss before serving.

LONG SAUTEED VEGETABLES

Ingredients:

Root and/or round vegetables such as onions, cabbage, carrots or parsnips cut into large pieces, 1/2 to 1 inch thick

Light sesame oil

Sea salt

Shoyu

Note: A cast iron skillet or heavy pan works best. No lid is needed.

Preparation:

- Heat the skillet, then add a little oil.
- Spread the oil evenly and heat it on a low flame.
- If using onion, sauté it first.
- Then add the firmest vegetable and sauté it until it is evenly coated with oil.
- Add a pinch of sea salt.
- Sauté all the vegetables over a low flame for 10 - 20 minutes or until they become tender.
- When needed, add a little water to prevent the vegetables from sticking to the pan.
- Towards the end of cooking, lightly season with shoyu and cook for another 4 - 5 minutes.

Option:

Sauté for half the time, add a little water and cover. Then simmer until the vegetables are tender. Season as above.

PRESSED SALAD or COLESLAW

Ingredients:

Head cabbage (round, green cabbage)

Celery

1 carrot

Sea Salt

Ratio: 1/4 - 1/2 teaspoon of sea salt per 4 to 5 cups of vegetables

Dressing Ingredients:

2 - 3 teaspoons of tahini

Several drops of shoyu

Preparation:

- Slice the vegetables very finely.

- Sprinkle in a small amount of sea salt and mix really well until the vegetables begin to sweat. The more thoroughly the pressed salad is mixed, the less salt is needed.

- Place in a bowl and fit a plate that is a bit smaller than the bowl on top of the vegetables. Place a heavy enough weight on top of the plate so that the vegetables are pressed down firmly. (A jar of beans works well.)

- Press at least 2 - 2 1/2 hours, no longer than 3 hours.

- Mix the dressing ingredients with chopsticks or a whisk, then dilute the mixture with a small amount of hot bancha tea or spring water. The dressing should be creamy, but not too thick. Add some brown rice vinegar for a sour taste.

- Remove the pressed vegetables from the bowl and drain off any excess liquid.

- Dress the salad and place in another serving bowl.